ROADS TO MEANING AND RESILIENCE WITH CANCER

Forty Stories of Coping, Finding Meaning,
and Building Resilience While Living
with Incurable Lung Cancer

Morhaf Al Achkar, MD, PhD

Dedication

To an angel with broken wings.

Acknowledgements

I want to express my gratitude for the love and care, my dad, Ahmad; my fiancée, Crystal; and my siblings, Bassem, Wafa, Hana, Nada, Amal, Malack, Houda, and Mustafa have all given me.

This work would not have been possible without the help and support of my oncologists, Laura Chow and Christina Baik; my friends, Kelly Davies, Marcel Shehwaro, Bill Philips, Malaz Boustani, Debra Revere, Dan Evans, Laura-Mae Baldwin, Matthew Thompson, Lu Marchand, Devon Elise, Elizabeth McKinnon-Somm, Gregory Sadler, Sizan Ava; and my mentor Phil Carspecken; and many others.

I want to thank Upal Basu Roy, Janet Freeman-Daily, Jill Feldman, Ivy Elkins, and Tom Carroll, for helping connect me to research participants. I also thank the ROSOneder support group, the ALK-Positive Facebook Support Group, and the EGFR Resisters for supporting and promoting this work. Thank you especially to all the 39 research participants who gave me the privilege to have conversations with them.

Table of Contents

For this consciousness has been fearful, not of this or that particular thing or just at odd moments, but its whole being has been seized with dread; for it has experienced the fear of death, the absolute Lord. In that experience it has been quite unmanned, has trembled in every fiber of its being, and everything solid and stable has been shaken to its foundations. But this pure universal movement, the absolute melting-away of everything stable, is the simple, essential nature of self-consciousness, absolute negativity, pure being-for-self.

— Georg Wilhelm Friedrich Hegel
"Phenomenology of Spirit."

Preface

I was driving back home from the lung doctor's office. He had tapped a couple of liters of fluids from around my lungs. Yes, it was painful. It felt as if someone was stabbing my back with a knife. It is as if you know that a sharp object is penetrating through the layers of your skin and muscles, but you also know you need to stay still and not resist it. When your lung expands is when it hurts the most.

Those airways had collapsed for so long under the pressure of the fluids around the lung that when they opened up again, I felt a pain like I never had before. I thought I couldn't take another breath. The pain and inability to breath lasted for only a few minutes, but it felt like hours.

After finishing the procedure, I headed home. That was the second time I'd had this fluid tap; the first was at the emergency room a few days before. As I was driving, I asked myself when this was going to end. I thought of the x-ray image of my shrunken lung and all the fluids around it and wondered when I would be back to my old self.

It turned out that would never happen.

Two days after I'd had those thoughts, I sat down with the same lung doctor in his office. He appeared concerned, and his face was dark. He still maintained a kind but faint smile of genuine care as he suggested that we go over the images of my chest that had been taken a few days prior. He explained what we were seeing.

Since I had looked at them myself, multiple times, and read the report, there was no news. But afterward, he went on to explain the results of the pathology report. He promised that he had called the pathologist himself to confirm them and that he had been shocked to find that there were "malignant cells in the fluid around the lungs."

It was cancer!

I knew that finding malignant cells in the fluids around the lung means a Stage 4 cancer of some sort. That is not good.

I have cancer, and it's Stage 4.

That was my first thought. But what I said first with my eyes starting to water was, "I am not an exception."

People get cancer, and I am one of the people.

I am also a family doctor, and throughout my career, I have taken care of people with cancer. I have ordered the workup for patients who presented with troubling symptoms and then given them the diagnosis of a malignancy. I had shared the news of difficult diagnoses with patients.

To think that I would have been immune from that same fate was not something to occur to me; anyone can develop cancer.

Still, when *you* are the one who has developed cancer, you are alone.

Your cancer is *your* disease, and while it can spread in your body, it fortunately does not spread to other people; the disease is isolating.

All of a sudden, your life path, which was once in parallel with the paths of others, takes a different turn. But you are still a person. You want to connect with others, and you want to share because what you experience is meaningful, at least to you. It is significant to you, and you wonder if others would see it the same way.

———————

I grappled for a long, long time with why to write about my experiences. I started writing a book at least four times.

But I have never finished the work.

When you write about yourself, some tensions and conflicts arise. Whenever I start writing, I struggle with the tension between writing about myself for me, as an authentic person, and writing for others in a way that is meaningful to them. There is also the guilt that arises because, as I tell my story, I become self-indulgent, and that is shameful.

Cancer patients, aware of their mortality, are sensitive to the vanity of self-indulgence.

It was not until November 2017, when a year had passed since my diagnosis, that the feelings became more mixed. There was the joy of still being alive after having thought I would be dying in a few months.

There was also the hope that comes with surviving one year: if I had survived 365 days, I could survive many more.

As I attempted to begin writing something about my experience, I found an article in a medical journal that led me to a whole body of work about the experience of lung cancer patients.

At first, I was scared to dive deeper into the struggle of others. A lot of the lung cancer patients described in the literature had died quickly. Many, with advanced diseases, did not have the opportunity to make sense of their story, let alone share it with others.

What troubled me the most, however, was that much of what had been written about the experiences of these patients had been written *about* the patients and not *by* them.

What was written about lung cancer patients was in a language I would not use to describe my own experience, as a subject with agency. There were words about the experiences of shame, blame, and guilt. There were also words about living in constant fear or in denial. They were words that one would use only when describing the experience of another that they, themselves, had never understood.

Because I struggled to understand my experience and make it understood to others, I thought I could do something here, and it became my commitment to lend my voice to the people who struggle with this illness.

I know how to have a conversation with people. I have learned as a doctor, and as a researcher, how to invite others into spaces of reflection and authentic dialogue. Should I not use my talent where I could make an impact?

That is why I decided to write this book.

I interviewed thirty-nine people with lung cancer, and in this book, I share aspects of our stories. They are individuals, like me, who are fortunate to be alive at a time when science has made it possible to survive with advanced lung cancer for more than a few months.

They are also like you, before their illness, men and women with busy lives, families, and friends. Some worked as doctors, teachers, writers, builders, and managers. Others stayed home to take care of their loved ones. Their ages ranged between thirty and seventy-five.

We are living longer than we initially expected, and this has made our experiences resemble nothing that many of us have lived or witnessed before.

These are authentic people who have had time to reflect and think about themselves and their lives in the face of the absolute dread: death. Many of them have captured with their words some of the essences of our struggles as humans. Some are examples to those who are curious about the meaning of our existence.

———————————

So, who am I writing this work to and for? I am writing to you, the person who has not yet had lung cancer. I am also writing to you, the person who still has the privilege to live with health. I am also writing to the ones whose stories are not written here, those who would find the most meaning if they opened their souls to the experiences of those tarrying at the limits of time.

Of course, if you have developed lung or another type of cancer, or if you have struggled with an illness, you will find aspects of your story reflected here.

And importantly, if you have experienced a crisis of identity and how you conceptualize yourself, you will find aspects of your story here as well.

From these thirty-nine individuals, I have learned far more than I have through any reading or writing. By sharing their experiences, I am merely opening the space for them to teach others. They have a lot of wisdom, and they have a lot of access to knowledge of good things.

I am also writing this story, on their behalf, to all those who would listen to them.

I am hoping that by developing the language to explain our struggles as cancer patients, others can understand us better, and with that, also better understand themselves. Those who made their life commitment to providing care for individuals who are struggling will also find what can help them here.

In other words, I am writing to a broad audience of everyday people.

I am reminded that, while being a researcher and doctor, I am first and foremost a person. My cancer has made this aspect of my identity, being a person, more salient. And because that is on my mind, I have become a better doctor, a better researcher, and a better teacher.

I am writing to all of us so that we can see ourselves in others and reflect on human experiences. It is only when we have this genuine dialogue and critical reflection that we come to understand others and ourselves. The goal of this work is not to enumerate the diversity of conditions and choices of people living with lung cancer but to also help us all understand and make sense of their experiences. Having the conversation on these pages will, I hope, facilitate the development of language that will help people understand and be understood.

This work is not merely a narrative. I am not just telling stories. This is a reconstruction of experiences and finding meaning within them. You will not find forty individuals sharing about their lives, one person after the other. Rather, I focus on the essence of the human experience, which is similar for many people. But when individuals dealt with the subject matter differently, I also brought to focus this diversity of human positions.

I am sure someone will say, why does this matter?

Well, lung cancer is the leading cause of cancer deaths and the second most common type of cancer in the United States.[1] In 2019 alone, it is expected that 228,150 people will be diagnosed with lung cancer, and over 142,670 will die from this nasty disease.[2]

Lung cancer is common—and deadly.

A significant proportion of patients with lung cancer are diagnosed at advanced stages and have a survival rate of a few months.[2] In addition, patients with lung cancer experience a significant burden from more than just the disease itself and its related symptoms but also from the treatment and its complications and many side effects.[3]

But there are glimmers of hope.

Nowadays, lung cancer is recognized as a heterogeneous disease.[4]

That means it is not one disease with a similar course for everyone. Recent advances in identifying genetic mutations and targeted therapies have improved the prognosis of some groups of patients. These include patients with anaplastic lymphoma kinase (ALK) positive lung cancer, epidermal growth factor receptor (EGFR), and proto-oncogene tyrosine-protein kinase ROS1 (ROS1).

Many patients with Stage 4 lung cancer who have these mutations and who are fortunate to be on the right treatment may now live for a few years, on average, rather than only a few months. Therefore, living with advanced lung cancer is beginning to resemble living with other cancers, such as breast cancer, which are today treated as chronic diseases.

This is really exciting and important.

As these patients with oncogenic alterations live longer, we have started to think of the disease differently. Survivorship is becoming a focus of attention. This is how the landscape of cancer care has changed in the recent years for many other cancers, and it is now shifting for lung cancer as well.

What has become relevant are issues related to the day-to-day lived experiences of the patient.[5,6] Because this new group of lung cancer survivors used to literally die in a few months and are now living for perhaps a few years, not much is known about the experience of extra years that they would never have had if they had contracted their cancer just five or ten years ago.

I am curious about those people, and I am also one of them. That is why I am doing this work. I have the purpose of sharing the stories of patients with advanced lung cancer who are on these targeted therapies so that we can learn together about their experiences in making meaning, building resilience, and dealing with the struggle that comes with this disease.

————————

How did I do this work?

I interviewed lung cancer patients to learn about different aspects of their experiences. The thirty-nine other participants (I am the fortieth) all had advanced or metastatic non-small-cell lung cancer with an oncogenic alteration (ALK, EGFR, ROS1), and they were all living and receiving care in eighteen different states in the United States.

I connected with these patients through lung cancer online support groups for patients, survivors, and caregivers. I sought their participation by announcing my research project and connecting with active members of these communities, who encouraged patients to participate.

We did the interviews either in person, by phone, or using videoconference. Each interview lasted about sixty to ninety minutes. I audio recorded the conversations, and the recordings were transcribed.

All the interviews started with questions on demographics and cancer characteristics. Then we covered five topics: life before the cancer diagnosis; diagnosing and treating the cancer; how the person was coping with the disease; life after the diagnosis; and, finally, their unmet needs.

I am a qualitative researcher and have a PhD in research methodology. I used robust qualitative methods to analyze the data concurrently with collecting the transcripts of interviews.[7] I described the methods of analysis in detail in a paper I have already written with a group of colleagues. Together, we explored the unmet needs and how we should improve these patients' experiences with health care.

In our completed study, we identified that

- Patients struggled to have meaningful lives while needing to work, manage finances, and navigate insurance. These patients needed understanding, emotional support, and extra practical assistance.

- Patients wanted their disease to be viewed and treated as a chronic condition, which gives them hope and aligns the focus of management of the disease with their goals.

- To improve their health care experience, patients wanted to have trust in their health care team, and they wanted to be engaged in conversations with health care providers as partners who are approached holistically as people.

In this book, I am building on that previous work and giving the space to the patients so they can tell more about how they find meaning, build resilience, and cope with this disease.

As you read this book, we will first go through how people with lung cancer find meaning. Then we will explore how they develop resilience and maintain strength in the face of this adversity. In the third part, we'll explore some health actions, what they are doing and why they are doing it. The fourth part is on coping in terms of finding ways to deal with the stress and the struggle.

I will share reflections from my own experience throughout as well.

It is important here to note that these stories are of people with lung cancer who have developed diseases unrelated to smoking. I am borrowing their privilege to call out the nonsense of the stigma around lung cancer as it relates to smoking.

People with lung cancer still feel stigmatized because of the association of their illness with tobacco use. I am one of them; I feel the stigma around my disease, and this is not right. I have not smoked, and yet I got lung cancer, and that is the case for most of the participants in this work.

I am taking the opportunity to call attention to the need for more research and support for lung cancer patients, whether or not they have ever smoked.

Part one:

FINDING MEANING

H

ow do you find meaning?

That is how I asked the question, and the participants gave their answers. There are many ways to learn about how a person finds meaning. You can look at how they spend their life and examine their work. You can also have conversations with them about different matters and infer from what they say about their frames of references and about what they find meaningful or relevant.

I chose to ask how the person finds meaning simply, like that.

There is no set way to think about the meaning of meaning. But people still consider this concept relevant to them, or at least many did. I wanted to ensure that people who did not think about concepts like meaning were still included in this narrative and reconstruction. And I was afraid that if I asked the question in any other way, I would be bringing out more of my own framework of meaning than anything about the others' thoughts.

Participants were in different places in their experiences and reflections. Some felt they had little access to purpose and meaning, as if it had all been ripped off from them or that life was nothing but chaos. Some also struggled in trying to reconcile any notion of fairness they had about life. It did not make sense for some that they, out of the many, were the ones who were suffering.

Some were still searching for peace and considered meaning to be a work in progress.

There was also a group of participants who reached beyond this life and found meaning there. They were the ones who found meaning in religion.

Others could not find comfort in faith and, instead, worked up something else. Among them, there was a group who sought knowledge and understanding in the working of humans, whether that is in science or the humanities. For some, this life was their only shot.

Many individuals found meaning in relationships and connections—those who had children or families connected with them to make memories. People also found communities where they felt a sense of belonging. Cancer became a foundation for a community of support and advocacy groups. The friends or family of cancer survivors became a reason for some individuals to carry on.

Those who were fortunate enough to return to work found meaning in the spaces where they showed their talents. Those who reconstructed their identities around their experience with cancer also found meaning in serving others, especially the ones who struggle with a similar illness. For them, meaning had become about service, and service gave them a purpose.

Not everyone, however, thought about their lives within a framework of meaning. Some simply lived their life and did not feel they needed to have an elaborate philosophy.

I relate to the many experiences of searching for meaning or purpose. The existential fear of death has provoked in me many questions about life and its meanings all at once. At some point, I wished that there would be an answer that I could reach out and grab with my hands. I could not, however, find that one answer. So I asked the thirty-nine people about their experience with meaning because I did not personally know the answer.

I am still on the search.

Not Finding the Meaning

At the center of the painting, a man is kneeling next to the lips of a statue of a sphinx. The man is wearing a cloth robe that covers most of his body except the left side of his chest and his left arm. He leans with his ears toward the sphinx, as if listening to it whisper. But the sphinx's lips are sealed.

The attentiveness in the man's posture tells that the sphinx was anything but generous with wisdom.

The man is standing on sand that extends, along with old ruins, into the distance. Only the head of the sphinx can be seen; the body is buried in the sand, as are the pillars and ruins. Next to the man is a stick he probably used to help him trudge through the sand so he could question the sphinx. In the right corner are a skull and a rectangular structure that looks like a tomb.

It was December of 2016, two weeks after I was diagnosed with Stage 4 lung cancer. I was in Boston, seeking a second opinion from Harvard and wandering through the Museum of Fine Art looking for meaning. I was staring at the painting of the *Questioner of the Sphinx* (by Elihu Vedder, 1836–1923).

Although my medical questions had all been answered, I left the city, like the questioner of the sphinx, with only more existential questions. The most urgent question I had was about the meaning of my life, especially now that it appeared to have been shortened.

How do other people find meaning?

I know the question is problematic, but it is relevant. Problematic because we may not have two people agreeing on the meaning of the word "meaning"; and relevant because we use the reference to meaning every day as if it is essential to our existence.

When I asked the thirty-nine participants in my study about meaning, they referred to something. The words meant something to them.

They had answers. Even those who said they didn't have any answers had answers.

I struggled with the question, and I knew I was not alone in my struggle.

Donna, a thirty-seven-year-old woman, framed the issue in her way. She understood the meaning in the sense of purpose, and cancer made her rethink purpose on an individual level, as a person. Donna had lost what she once thought was her purpose in life. "How to find meaning? Hmm. That's a tough one," Donna remarked. "Cancer has forced me to focus and reflect on what's my purpose in life."

Donna had a sense of what having a purpose *had* been like. "I have a 9-year-old niece, and I had always thought that my purpose in life was to have a child of my own." But when Donna was diagnosed with cancer, that purpose was no longer attainable. "So, it's as if my purpose in life was ripped away from me," she said.

She has to be on the anticancer medication the rest of her life, and with that, she cannot biologically have a child of her own because the medicine would cause congenital abnormalities in her offspring. Therefore, even if she were to live another twenty years, it would not change the fact that she would not have biological children of her own. So now Donna is trying to find a purpose somewhere else, but she does not yet know what that is.

Stories of finding meaning in the illness are known to survivors. But unless the person experiences the epiphany themselves, all those stories are just words.

There was Nancy, a thirty-six-year-old woman, for instance. She rejected the notion that she found meaning anywhere in her experience with cancer. "I don't think I have found meaning; I don't think I have," she responded. "I think if anything, this just reinforced to me the idea that life is just chaos and that there is no purpose to things."

Nancy perceived that she'd had a significant derailing of her life path. Although many people came to console her by bringing their reasonings or understandings of the world, she could not find condolences in their words. Nancy heard people say, "Just let go," and "Everything happens for a reason." But these did not fit with how she saw things.

You know, no! No! There are horrible, horrible things that happen in this world, absolutely atrocious, way worse than what has happened to me. And they didn't happen for a reason.

Nancy could not relate to an understanding that finds a reason for everything that happens. She could not let go of calling things what they are. Things can be ugly, and that sucks. Life sucks at times and for no reason. So Nancy could not find meaning. "I don't think I found it—I haven't found any meaning in it. If anything, it's that life is very fleeting."

Nancy was not alone in her position. Sandra had a similar experience, although she was more open to one day finding meaning, as others do. Sandra explained, "I read about these people who say that now is the time to make memories and live because you don't know what's going to happen." However, she did not easily relate.

I'm not there yet. I'm still kind of battling the sadness and feel like the things that I had in my life have been taken away from me. So I'm trying to get to where maybe I can eventually see that life is special and precious. And I've had a scare, so enjoy things now because you don't know what the future holds. But I'm just not there yet; working on it.

Sandra saw that some people do come to terms with this, yet this acceptance was not yet attainable for her. Sandra hoped it would come with time, although when she looked inward, she realized she was still battling an endless sadness. Maybe someday, she hoped, she would get to a place where she could find peace.

For some, the question of fairness still haunted. Fairness is another notion that is relevant to a conceptualization of meaning, or to at least having a framework that makes things make sense.

Just like Sandra, who thought things had been taken away from her, David, a forty-two-year-old man, felt the magnitude of the loss and believed it was not fair. David explained,

I feel it's unfair. I don't understand. I'm a Catholic, and I used to go to church a lot. I don't understand how God could do this to me. Why would He give me this? What have I done? Why do I deserve this?

Cancer has shaken David's faith, but he still keeps on with it. He explains, "I stopped praying for a while, and just now, I am coming more to terms with it. I started praying again. But I still feel it's unfair, and I don't understand why this happened to my family and me."

To David, it was simply unfair. At least at first, he could not make sense of it. It was not what he had expected, and that wasn't right. Still, he did what he could to keep holding on to something.

Similarly, Christine, a forty-five-year-old female, continued to grapple with the question of why me, and when I asked about finding meaning, she said, "I don't find meaning. I don't know. I say stuff like why. Why me? All that stuff. I will look for meaning. I haven't found it yet."

Just like David, who at times comes closer to accepting yet goes back to asking the same question, so did John. He also considered his search for meaning to be an unfinished task.

John, a thirty-two-year-old, thought his purpose was to promote a healthy diet so people could live disease free. But in the middle of giving one of his talks to people about how diet prevents cancer, he could not use his voice anymore. He was diagnosed with lung cancer. Now, he is back to searching for meaning, and he explains,

> I'm still trying to figure it out. It's still—I guess it's a work in progress, and it changes. It's constantly changing. You know, before, I thought my purpose was to help people get healthy through nutrition by using my technique of meal prepping and making it easy for them, making it convenient.

His illness tested the limits of his frame of reference. Does diet prevent cancer? If it doesn't, then what was he doing? What was his life about?

What cancer did not test in him, however, was the desire to do things with others and for others. He explains, "Now, I'm starting to think maybe that it's helping people with cancer and helping people who are already ill get better through nutrition. So I don't know." He still insists on helping people to get better nutrition. Maybe nutrition does not completely prevent cancer, but maybe it can help with healing. One thing that has not changed for him is finding meaning in helping people.

It is an unanswered question. In response to my questions, Nancy said, later in our conversation,

> The only meaning that I could come up with is that life is precious, and I'm trying to enjoy it as much as I can. We should experience it while we're here and be present in it and try to live a life that makes the world a better place before you leave it.

Life is precious, and even though the world can be an ugly place, it can also be made better. Life is an unfinished project, and similarly, finding meaning is an uncompleted task.

That is what I learned about struggling to find meaning, and that is what the sphinx in Boston had not told me.

The Meaning Is There All Around

I shared with a friend about my plan to write this book. He was skeptical. Maybe I shared with him because I knew he would be skeptical. I needed a voice of doubt and wisdom. I shared that one of my most important tasks with this book was to explore how people grapple with meaning. I also reflected on my position in regard to the matter.

I was concerned that in writing a book about others' struggle with meaning, I may actually be writing a book about my own. Maybe that is why I had doubts and wanted his skepticism. I worried that the existential restlessness of others that I was exploring was simply a reflection of my struggles with the matter, which I'd had even before the illness.

He was concerned that these questions had been tackled for centuries by philosophy and religion. So what was there to add? He also worried because of my position on the matters of faith and religion. How can one person step out of their frame of reference to truthfully represent that of others?

I explained that while I was raised Muslim, I am now agnostic, and I have taken an open position to learn about the values brought to the conversation by all frames of references. I also realize that there are elaborate philosophies and major religions out there that have presented all-encompassing frameworks for thinking about life as a whole. And I confess that I come here with skepticism about the possibility of maintaining a religious view that is coherent and consistent with modern views of the world.

However, I accept that people are entitled to their religious position and their spiritual aspirations. The individual can look at the list of options and choose for themselves. Or they can choose to not look and simply take in whatever comes their way. That does not trouble me in any way. I am only curious about how the person of faith experiences this illness. I was interested in hearing their stories and how those stories came to be. I was curious to understand and was open to the differences.

I present here the views of those who referenced faith or reflected on their relationship with religion.

I was privileged to learn about Kim's view of life. Kim's frame of reference included the notion that everyone has their struggle. Her system of thought explains that to her well, and she finds that makes sense. She shared with me,

> One of our Catholic beliefs is that everyone has a cross to bear. So, I've looked at it as this happens to be the one that I've been asked to bear. I also offer up my suffering to Jesus. That's another Catholic belief. We're taught that we are offering up our suffering or sharing in Jesus's suffering through our suffering.

Kim is mindful of the suffering she is experiencing, and she is not taught to deny it.

Her suffering is emotional, as she explained. "I've physically been OK. Now, I've gone through some treatments that were not super fun but nothing debilitating. But the suffering has been more emotional or psychological." For her, that counts as suffering, the same as any physical pain or bodily struggle. Her suffering is also not wasted. It is instead part of her journey on a higher path. She explained that "suffering is like a path to holiness."

Also, within her framework, her suffering is like a test. Kim said, "God is testing me, testing my faith. So one of the things I pray for is that. Other than praying for healing, I pray that my faith remains strong because it's times like these that your faith can really falter." Within this framework, maintaining faith is how to pass the test.

I see how suffering can be framed neutrally, "We all suffer, and this is my fair share," or even positively as "an offer to Jesus and as an opportunity." Also—and here is the concern of the believer—"as a test, the person could fail." Failing the test by losing faith is the worst of it all. Kim explained it this way: "The suffering for me is not the physical, because I have been physically fine, but is the emotional suffering and, more importantly, the questioning."

It is the doubt that sneaks into the heart of the person who suffers that is the real suffering, Kim added. "The questioning of why did this happen? How could God let this happen to me? I thought I did all the right things, and still, this happened to me, and the unfairness of it all." However, Kim recognizes that she is not the only one suffering. She goes to a support group and sees others who are struggling. She says,

> There are a lot of much younger patients than I am and I just think, "Gosh, I thought I was young," and then I hear about all these other people who are much younger.

The real suffering is in the question that does not find answers. But Kim does not let those concerns take her all the way, which she reminds herself.

> But then again, I have always to trust that there's a plan for me, and it's out of my control, so I'm not in charge. I always have to just go back to that, and if suffering happens to be part of the plan, then I have no choice but to accept it.

For Kim, the individual is not in charge. It is God who is in charge. God is in charge, and He has a plan.

Kim was fifty years old when we had our conversation, and at that time, she'd had her illness for seven months. She was married, with two college-age children. She had been a stay-at-home mom for most of the past eighteen years, although she had recently been considering reentering the workforce.

Born in the United States, Kim had spent most of her childhood in the Philippines. Her husband, about three years older, had been the primary breadwinner of the family for the last eighteen years, since their second child had been born. That's when she had decided she was better off staying at home and raising her family than working outside the home.

In the months leading up to the diagnosis, she had been settling into a new routine as a recent empty nester; they had just sent their youngest off to her freshman year at college. Once her kids had gone away to college, she started looking for jobs. But being out of the job market for so long made it harder to find one. Then she accepted a job offer only a few weeks before her diagnosis of advanced and inoperable lung cancer. She would be working at a Catholic school in the area. Her efforts to find a job had come to fruition, but the diagnosis put a damper on that job offer. To her, it meant that God had a different plan.

For Amy, also, God has the plans and gives meaning in life. For her, that matter is clear. She said, "There is God; there is divine intervention." Amy was sixty-three years old when we had our conversation, and she had been diagnosed for about four and a half years. Amy sold commercial real estate, and her husband was a surgeon when the couple had decided to take early retirement. They had a weekend house in the countryside that became their home. A few years before her diagnosis, a few lung nodules had been found on an x-ray. She was having regular imaging studies to make sure the nodules were not malignant. After about a year and a half of keeping an eye on the spots, during which she'd kept hearing that was nothing to worry about, her surgeon husband had asked, "Why are you subjecting yourself to so much radiation, because that can cause cancer, you know?" She started to worry, "and I just acquiesced and decided to stop going for scans."

Then she had a car accident. She explains that, in her mind, it was "divine intervention about ten months after I'd had my last scan." Amy had been driving on twisty country roads in a light rain. When a car approached from the opposite direction, she seemed to have overcompensated and hit a rock to the side. Amy's car flipped over and was totaled. Amy was taken to a trauma center not far away, where they scanned her and then said, "You have a broken back and lung cancer."

Amy is Jewish, and since she was a teenager, she has been part of a synagogue. She believes in God and divine intervention. She believes in one god with many interpretations. Amy says she always wished to find, wherever she was, a place of worship that was "open to all religions and is a spiritual church. And that's the kind of place I would like to be."

Amy explains, "If I didn't have that car accident, I probably would have been diagnosed later with Stage 4 (she was first diagnosed with Stage 3b and then progressed to 4), and God knows if I would've ever been diagnosed at all. I could've died in my sleep. Either I got suffocated or who knows? I had a large tumor. But I feel that I'm meant to be here."

She hears that from other people as well. People enjoy her presence and the thoughtfulness she brings, and they often tell her things like, "I'm so glad that you were in my life today. I'm so glad that I had the opportunity to help you," or "I'm so glad that we hear your thoughts." She feels she is here for a purpose. Now, with her experience with cancer, and with her faith, she hears things differently than before. For Amy, the meaning is there, and it is all around.

It is an eternal meaning, and it has always been.

No Major Philosophies

I may not live for much longer, and I need to know the Truth. Not this or that truth, but *the Truth!*

That was how I felt in the period immediately following my diagnosis. I had pushed the significant questions about the meaning of life to the side while I had been busy living and learning. But now I didn't have much time left to defer those questions anymore.

The urgency was immense.

I wished there was one way to know. I wished there was something that would take me to Truth like a shot from a pistol, to use Friedrich Hegel's words. I wanted that kind of path to truth: fast and secure. Having urgency does not, however, change the rules of knowing.

Just because the person wants to know and wants to know now does not make this knowledge happen. If anything, with the urgency comes hurried attempts at understanding, and those are often blind or misguided. I had the belief that because I had little time left, I needed to find the masterpieces of humanity's work. I needed to take them in so I would understand more.

Many would argue that philosophy reached its peak with Hegel, who is my second favorite philosopher, so I picked up *Phenomenology of Spirit*. In the book, Hegel lays out the stages Spirit moves through on its path to Absolute Knowledge. And that is what I wanted—to know the Absolute. I thought if I could traverse this path, I would arrive at knowing.

I read the book once, then twice, and then five times. In the end, Hegel disappointed me. He did not give me what I was after, Truth. However, he did liberate me from many old habits of the mind, such as the search for a mysterious path to knowing. Upon reflection, he also freed me of my futile pursuit itself! Hegel taught me that it is only with labor and by tarrying with the negative through a formative experience that I could know more.

Hegel also saved my life. If rather than picking up *Phenomenology*, I had picked up a book of faith, I would probably have been in a different place.

I wonder now what I would be writing here in that parallel reality. I can imagine that I would probably be writing "(fill in the blank) saved my life." We often have certainty in what we believe regardless of whether or not it has truth.

Hegel saved me, but those who read Hegel understand that you can get lost in the dialectics. Are all those opposites the same? I would say no, they are not. If I did not find Truth in the end, is this word, truth, even meaningful? Yes, the word truth is meaningful, and there is better truth. I learned that, however, not from Hegel, but from another philosopher named Jürgen Habermas.

Habermas, a German philosopher, is my favorite philosopher of all time. He is still alive and just turned ninety. And he continues to be one of the most influential philosophers of our age. I had a dream once that I was having coffee with him, and we were chatting about philosophy. I asked him about my third favorite philosopher, Emanuel Kant, and whether we can still view as valid what Kant had said about the impossibility of knowing God in himself.

Habermas did not answer, and the dream ended.

I wish I could have coffee with Habermas, and I am writing that in this book so that maybe he will read it and help make it happen.

With Habermas, I came to realize that I will not be able to have a philosophy that makes sense of everything. I will not find a system that can explain everything once and for all. While Habermas was not the first to say that, he was, for me, the first to elaborate a framework of understanding that was urgently needed.

While I may not reach the truth, I can continue to work toward understanding others. Habermas gave me a framework for judging truth, rightness, and authenticity. I needed that framework to have these conversations with others and to know about myself and about them. I need it still so that I can seek better truth, better rightness, and more authenticity.

I reflect now and wonder if I would still be able to live with meaning without those elaborate frameworks. Do we still need philosophy?

Other participants chose not to explain meaning by referring to major systems of philosophy or religion. This is where James came from when he reflected, "I do not have any great amazing philosophies about life after death." For him, it is merely this life and only this life.

Ashes to ashes, and dust to dust.

James did not want to go for meaning that is beyond the immediate. As he puts it, "I just want to be around for as long as I can to continue helping others and enjoying life myself, which I do." James loves traveling, photography, playing chess, kayaking, and hiking, and he does lots of things that he enjoys. He recognized that some might see this as shallow, but that is all right. James would accept the argument that people are just shallow, and he did not want to go into this "old discussion."

James was then sixty years old, and when he was diagnosed, he was fifty-seven. He had been a dentist since the age of twenty-one, first in Australia and then in the United States, and had retired. He had enjoyed doing dentistry for patients who needed dentistry. He saw clientele from a low or middle socioeconomic demographic. "It wasn't like cosmetic dentistry," he said. Rather, his work was "functional dentistry that needed doing." In other words, as he put it, "I wasn't doing bullshit dentistry." It was good, gratifying work, and he has no regrets about it.

James is also an immigrant who did and still does good things for the community, whether in his work life as a dentist serving those in need or in his retirement, when he leads work in advocacy and support groups. For him, you do not need major philosophies to explain why this is good and right; you can do it without thinking much about what it means.

Brandon did not find an easy answer to the question about meaning either. He said, "That's a hard question," and then he went silent for a while before pointing out that people may think things happen deliberately for them or to them, but that was not how he saw the world.

> I guess I don't really look too hard for meaning. I don't feel like anything that happens to me, whether it's good or bad, is something that someone or something has deliberately meant for me or has done to me. I don't know. I don't know if I really look too hard for meaning in things, if that makes any sense.

It did make sense. Brandon was forty-eight years old when we talked, and he'd had the disease for seventeen months. He is married to his wife of eighteen years, and they have two daughters. At the time of his diagnosis, their daughters were sixteen and thirteen. He worked full time in the logistics industry. He has a bachelor's degree in international relations with Spanish as his major, and he also has a master's of international economics and management he competed in Italy at a graduate school in Milan. He explained

> My upbringing was a little bit different in the sense that both
> of my parents were diplomats for the State Department. So,
> in my childhood, we moved like every two or three years to a
> different country, to a different posting. So we moved around
> a lot.

He grew to love traveling because he experienced different places and different cultures. When you travel around the world, you can find yourself invisible in an ocean of people. You then tend to see the world as having a reality and rules of its own, rules that often do not revolve around the person. It is hard, then, to maintain a view of the world that is centered on yourself. And having no such view can liberate you from the desire to explain things as intended for or directed at you personally.

Living in a foreign land can liberate one from viewing oneself as the center of the meaning of everything that happens around them. Things happen, for us or without us, and we are just there.

Not very far from this was Emily's position. For her, life's fairness is not about the person being immune to experiencing adverse circumstances. Emily puts it this way:

> I don't think life is fair. I think that people get sick and that
> · people have adversity. Yes, people don't always get to be as
> healthy as they would wish to be, and people have a lot of stuff
> like cancer as well.

Emily is a forty-six-year-old humanities professor who was diagnosed four months before our interview. She is married to another professor, of humanities and literature, and together, they have two boys who were eleven and fourteen at the time. They live in a college town that is "very typical upper middle class in the sense of a privileged sort of life." Life for Emily had been about balancing her work in research, the kids, service, and her students. Her hobbies are cooking and "lazy gardening." She takes walks, and while not an athlete, she is physically active. She bikes for transportation, describing herself as "extremely environmentally conscious." She also goes to the farmers' market, cooks vegetables, and has a sweet tooth.

Emily is aware of her privilege. Many people do not have what she has, and she learned to not take that for granted. She explains,

> I have cancer, and we've got so much going on, which is true. But I'm not worried, like, no one's turning off the light on me. I'm not losing my health insurance. My house is safe. Nothing's being repossessed. I'm not worried about the day-to-day. I'm not worried about my children's safety. So I'm worried about things like, "Oh no, this one didn't make the soccer team, and now he's kind of sad. I hope he joins the debate club." I'm not worried they're going to be unsafe.

She is aware that in this life, because we are human, people do get sick. If we view life from a social perspective, in her view, it is unjust not because people get ill but because there are people with privileges, and there are people with none. Looking at life as a part of nature means it is not about fairness. Things happen. Still, our society is not just or fair, and this social injustice could be something to call out as in need of change or as a reason to be angry.

Mary took another stab at the issue of thinking it's not fair. She looked around and found people with problems and struggles all over the place, and that made her think that "Everybody has their own shit that they deal with. My problems are not any better or any worse than what somebody else might have."

One may not be in a position to say it isn't fair if they listen to the stories of struggles that other people experience. I liked what Mary said, and it is not hard to see how much all people, we and others, struggle every day. The only exception would be to live with no adversities.

Mary is forty-six years old and was approaching her third year of survival when we she shared her story with me. She is married and has two boys. Six months before her illness, they were moving her oldest son into his dorm, and the family was getting used to life as a family of three instead of a family of four. Her youngest son was passionate about baseball, and their lives revolved around baseball at that time. She was a board member on their area's Little League.

She also worked full time as a commissions processor at a financial broker-dealer in the area. She had worked there for four years before her diagnosis, and she loved her job, especially "going into work, interacting with not only my coworkers but with the representatives that we got with through the financial industry." She saw herself as continuing to move up in her job. She was taking on more responsibilities and had gotten an excellent raise.

Being at a point in their lives where they were starting to think about what they wanted after their youngest left home, Mary and her husband made a plan that once their youngest son graduated from high school, they would put their house up for sale. "We wanted to live on a lake," she said. They were starting to do things around the house to get it updated before they put it up for sale. They lived in the house Mary had grown up in, and they had lived there for over seventeen years. Mary noted, "It was supposed to be our five-year home but ended up being our seventeen-year home."

Life does not always go as planned. But if we look around, is that not the case for everyone? You may not need elaborate philosophies to make sense of things. Philosophy can help, though, when we bring it down to the level of day-to-day conversations about understanding meaning.

Here, I am using "meaning" to refer to that which we understand. Meaning does not have to be elaborate, and philosophies do not have to make sense of everything at once. Science and modern philosophy have taught us to give up on understanding the totality of one system.

Still, someone can carry on with the idea that she needs or wants to carry on. And philosophy can help, although many individuals can do the job without sophisticated philosophies.

When we step out of seeing ourselves as the center of the system of reference, and when we compare our lives to others, it may be useful to avoid notions like fairness where there is no place for thinking of fairness.

It is absolutely not fair that some people have no access to health care. It is not fair that marginalized people cannot attain in life what people with privilege do. But this framework does not apply to cancer afflicting someone. As a random biological event, cancer can affect anyone, and it takes someone believing in their extreme exceptionality to justify feeling that they should not be affected by cancer when everyone else can be.

It is, however, fair to expect that we should be treated with care when we suffer. What is unfair is that people do not receive the care they need. And you do not need a major in philosophy to know that.

Meaning in Knowing

My mentor was skeptical when I told him that I was pursuing a PhD in Education. He said, "After you obtain a terminal graduate degree, people stop looking horizontally at the letters next to your name. They look vertically at the experiences you had and the work you did."

I could not argue against that. I still went for the degree.

My program of study was inquiry methodology in social science. The program is about learning how to methodically ask questions and how to research the matter at hand. The focus is on social sciences, and the emphasis is on the theory and practice of research. It is as much philosophical investigation as it is empirical questions.

At that time, I was struggling with a condition called inflammatory bowel disease. I was worried the disease could spin out of control and cost me part or all of my colon or that, with time, it could develop into cancer. As a physician, I was afraid that my illness could make it impossible for me to be a doctor, and I wanted to be prepared for a new identity.

What was most important is that I had the desire to know and understand. I was not, however, going after this or that specific piece of information; I simply wanted to know in general. I explained to my mentor that I was after an unknown answer to an unknown question, and I was hoping to find the question and search beyond what is known. He did not buy into that. But without that training in inquiry, I would not have been in a position to do the research that is the foundation of this book, and I would not have been in a place to talk to the people whose stories I share here.

What I learned in school, I have brought to bear in what I am now writing.

I interviewed people who also wanted knowledge and found meaning in it. For example, there is Lisa, who advocates that you do not need to be religious to think of meaning. Meaning for her has to do with *knowing*. She explained,

I have a tattoo on my back. It's my first one. I didn't get it until after my diagnosis, and it's straightforward. It's just a line that says, "All knowledge is worth having," and that's pretty much it.

That is the heart of it for Lisa. Meaning is in seeking knowledge. By that, she doesn't mean only one type of knowledge. She says, "I would never say that I have so much medical knowledge." She enjoys history. She enjoys anthropology. She is not religious in any way, but she explains, "One of my favorite subjects is comparative religion." She looks at it from an anthropological and cultural point of view, not so much a spiritual point of view. Lisa enjoys watching documentaries and shared, "I like comparing and finding meaning across cultural differences and through historical timelines." It is coming to know, and learning is the way to develop meaning.

Lisa was sixty-five years old, and she was one month shy of three years since her diagnosis when we had our conversation. Lisa had been diagnosed "in a year of transition." Everything came up quickly. Two years prior, she had been working at a job that had an intense commute, spending almost three hours in the car every day. She'd had the job as a literary sales manager for a newspaper for twenty-five years, but about two years before her diagnosis, the job started to fall apart. She said, "It was, of course, that Amazon took over everything."

She found herself a commission-only sales manager for a very well-known newspaper, but all the bookstores she worked with were going out of business. "My income plummeted from a very nice income to a very lousy income, and the company was starting to go under." Then, at that juncture, her mother, who'd had malignant melanoma, passed away. "They never found anything to help her; she died very quickly after diagnosis."

Her mother left a little bit of money, which allowed Lisa to quit her job, and she went back to school to pursue a certificate in health care advocacy. Her husband has a decent job, they had good health care, and her son was in college on a scholarship. "So, it was pretty easy to go ahead and just go to school." She got her certificate from a prestigious institute, then "everything happened at once," and that's when she was diagnosed.

Cancer, knowledge, and meaning all came together for Lisa.

Lisa is not the only one who found refuge not in faith but rather in books. Another participant who was in a similar position is Debora. Here, she explains:

> See, I'm not religious, and a lot of people get comfort from their religion, from believing in an afterlife and that once you die, everything is going to be fantastic, and you're going to see people and blah, blah, blah. I don't buy into that.

Instead, what Debora found helpful was bringing her attention to day-to-day subjects like "reading some books." Debora was sixty-four years old and had been diagnosed for a little over two years when we had our conversation. Her significant other is her high school sweetheart. Back in high school, they went together for about two and a half years. Through the years, they had kept in touch off and on. They had both married and had kids. She talked about when they got back together:

> So about ten years ago, he was divorced, I'm divorced, so we met for dinner, we start talking, we went on a trip together, what not, and then we became a couple. So we've been together for ten years; we have a good relationship and a good life.

Debora was a marketing manager for a big consulting firm that was going through a reorganization and merger. The company was downsizing, and Debora was in the middle of being laid off. When she learned about getting laid off, she was at first "pissed off," but then she thought it could be good because she would be getting out of a stressful job and would get an excellent severance package. In the end, things were good, and that was that.

Still, it is hard for her to accept that everything will always be fantastic or OK in the end. Her life has had many twists and turns that challenge such certainty and that *taught* her otherwise.

Not having faith does not mean the person would be suffering from uncertainty and constant doubts. For Cynthia, finding the meaning is not a struggle because she understands science. She explained,

I had never really struggled for meaning. I find it interesting enough through science and nature. Those are the things that give my life meaning. I'm not a religious person, so I don't have any faith-based support, and I don't believe in an afterlife. I don't believe in heaven or hell. I don't believe in any of that. I don't believe in God. So, really for me, it's all about the here and now and creating the most of what we have at the moment.

Cynthia was fifty-two, and she'd had her diagnosis for twenty-one months when we talked. In the years leading up to her diagnosis, she had divorced her husband, so it was just her and their three children. At the time of diagnosis, she was in a new relationship with a woman who is now her wife, and things were good.

She had gone back to work doing seasonal jobs, in the winter as a tax preparer, and in the summer, she'd recently returned to a previous career doing gardening and landscaping. She had "a nice balance." They were living in a new house and were very active and traveling frequently the year she was diagnosed.

Her frame of meaning-making had been tested before when she lost her mother to lung cancer. She shared,

> I was older than my children likely will be when they lose me, but I still feel the loss of her every day. Not in the way that's like it crippled me.

It is not loss that would make Cynthia sit in mourning or grieving because her mother is present in her life every day. Cynthia notices her mother in the things that she does, the things that she says, and the actions that she takes. "My mother is there when I wrap a Christmas present because she taught me how to do it so beautifully." It feels to her as if her mother is "moving through me every day."

When she imagines her children after she dies, she feels hopeful that she will also be with them. Cynthia explained, "So when I feel hope for the future and for my children, I feel that they're always going to have me with them as they go forward through life."

For Cynthia, you do not need this or that religious belief, and you do not need to know that you will be OK. What will happen to her has already been modeled when it happened to someone she loves—her mother.

Our lost ones still live with us in the memories we have here and now, not beyond this life.

The position on meaning, on life and what is beyond, and the interest in the here and now is salient also for Andrew. With the faith of a believer, Andrew asserts that there is nothing out there waiting for us. This is our one and only shot. He explained,

> I don't believe in an afterlife; I don't think there's something out there waiting for me in a better way after all of this. This is my one shot at the world.

This is not a position about a metaphysical question. For Andrew, this matter is relevant to day-to-day striving. He explained,

> I am going to try to maximize my time here, and that means I'm not lying down and taking this. This cancer is not going to take me quietly. I'm going to make every reasonable effort to stay alive, and that means doing drug trials and making sure I understand what the latest treatments mean and getting multiple stacks of opinions, as I have done, and continuing to see other doctors; just trying to stay out of the curb. So, that's one way I deal with it is to say I'm going to continue to fight, and I'm going to do it.

For Andrew, the matter ought to be taken into one's own hands. The questions are not theoretical but practical: what is it that I would do here and now? They are also not metaphysical but empirical questions: what is the best way to keep me alive and optimize my chances?

Andrew was sixty-one years old and had cancer for eleven months when we had our conversation. Until he was diagnosed, he was working for a computer company as one of two people running the legal department.

There were 500 people in his group. "So I had a big job; it was worldwide. I spent a lot of time traveling, a lot of time with legal issues." For over twenty years, his life was "very work focused." He was planning on retiring and had almost retired a few months prior, then chose to delay it, before he became ill and then had to retire.

Andrew is a subscriber to the *New England Journal of Medicine*, the journal with the greatest impact in medicine, so that he can have access to knowledge. He wants to be able to converse with his doctors, and more importantly, I think, he wants to know.

When we sense a boundary of time, our curiosity awakens, and so do our desires for knowledge.

It is with curiosity to know that we construct meaning.

Meaning in Being with Family

I received a wedding invitation a little over a year after my diagnosis. My nephew's wedding was planned for six months after the invitations were received. I wanted to be there, but six months is too far in advance to plan for someone with Stage 4 lung cancer.

Would I be here? Would I be strong enough to fly?

It is now months after the wedding, and they are pregnant. I made it to the wedding, and I am now looking at family photos. The couple gave the family a joyous reason to all get there and be together. I traveled the furthest, from Seattle to Malmerspach, a small town on the northeast side of France. I saw many of my relatives as well, some of whom had escaped the war in Syria. Like many of them, I did not take for granted that we were there.

It was good. It was a time to feel the community and family love. The memories will always be there, and so will the hundreds of photos. I was with my girlfriend at the time, now my fiancée, Crystal.

With family, there is unconditional care and love. When with family, all time is well spent. The family we are born into is not a personal choice. I came to life as the youngest of nine siblings. But my siblings have chosen to bring into this life, so far, twelve nephews and nieces. I have decided to be with Crystal, and I sought our love. The sufficient and necessary condition to love and be loved is to find someone who loves you and allows you to love them. That is what I believed, and for me, that was Crystal.

However, the question of having children is a difficult one and will always be a challenge. The child I could bring to life does not have a choice, and the moral burden is all mine. I will grapple with the notion as I have never had children and do not have any personal experience that resembles having my own. So the matter is not resolved or understood for me.

Among those who have children and families of their own, they find in them the most meaning. Linda explains how her children are the meaning of her life, although she had at first also been unsure how to answer the question about meaning. She explained,

What comes to my mind is that I have three kids. I didn't have meaning in my life before them; they are the meaning in my life. They're my motivation. They're the reason that I do things.

Linda was forty-one when we had the interview, and she'd had the diagnosis for thirty-two months. She has three girls and was diagnosed about a year after the birth of her third daughter. She described it, "So I still had a nursing baby when I was diagnosed. About a year before that, I was having a baby." When we talked, her daughters were five years, three years, and one year old.

Linda is a clinical psychologist by trade, and she has her own practice. She was happily married and "trying to manage the demands of three little kids" as well as her own business at the time of her diagnosis.

Regarding the kids, Linda says they are "wonderful, full of energy." The oldest is now going into the third grade. "She is not much of a student. She's not that interested in school, but she is all motor. She loves to play. She loves to run. She never stops moving, and she does anything that she can. Her big activity right now is that she does parkour, so she keeps us busy with her moving all around." Linda says that her second daughter "loves studying; she loves reading, and was a very proficient reader before she went to kindergarten and has always loved to just be in front of a book and learn everything that she can." And there is her baby. "The baby loves being a baby. I think she missed out on some of her babyhood because I was going through all that I was going through, and so now, everyone extra dotes on her, and she really appreciates it."

Things go by rapidly when kids are young, and the memories blur. Linda remarked, "You know, it's such a blur when you have little kids. It's all just sort of a mashup. My oldest has never really been a good sleeper, and so parents—we didn't get a lot of sleep, so it was a lot of just making it through the day. You know, getting the school lunches prepared and finding a way to get everyone dressed and out the door in the morning."

Linda enjoys a lot of family time and just snuggling. "We've always been a family that likes to sort of snuggle up on the couch and watch a movie or go to whatever sort of festival is there that day. We like to spend time together doing whatever it is that's available to us that day."

She met her husband about twenty years ago when they worked together. With Linda's cancer diagnosis, life for the couple has become "really just one day at a time."

Having children also made Elizabeth choose how to deal with her cancer. She wants to keep going because she wants her kids' memories of her to be good ones. She explained, "The kids are OK; and if the kids see me OK and that I'm doing stuff, they will be OK." Elizabeth has put effort into maintaining her children's lives as they were before her diagnosis. She told me, "Their lives haven't changed. They are getting to all their activities, and so everybody's OK."

She does not want to think about the illness and its prognosis. She explained, "You know, it doesn't help for me to dwell on what could happen and how long I have because I don't know how long I have. Nobody knows how long I have. I know that I have a lot of hope about the mutation I have and who knows?" She had just met a fourteen-year survivor with her same mutation. "So who knows? And I'm not even at year one yet. I haven't even gone there, and I have no idea what's gonna happen, so I need to keep going and keep their lives whatever they are right now." Elizabeth also puts effort into making sure the memories are positive. She said, "I want their memories to be of me living with it and going on, so I want their memories of me to be good ones and not of me in bed and sad that I had cancer."

Elizabeth was forty-three years old when we talked, and she'd had her diagnosis for twelve months. She was an airline pilot but had stopped working over a decade earlier due to an unrelated medical situation. She was a mom of two children and prided herself for living in a supportive community. Before her cancer diagnosis, she was very active with her kids and in the school and their community.

Her eight-year-old son has high functioning autism, and Elizabeth is very involved with his life, his therapies, and all of his needs. She also has a one-year-old daughter who is "typical developing." Her husband, also an airline pilot, is home half the month, "and then he's gone half the month. So he works a week and then he's away the whole time, and then he comes home for a week, and then he's away for a week, and then he's home for a week." Her life had been revolving around the kids before cancer, and it became even more about them after the diagnosis.

Having a family got some participants into a specific frame of mind as it relates to their emotions. Michael voiced it, "I'm not afraid to die; I'm afraid not to live." That would not have been the case for Michael if he did not have his son. His son is an inspiration and a reason to be alive. He elaborated,

> Well, I think my frame of mind would certainly be different if my son weren't here. Without him knowing it, he is my main inspiration. I want to see him grow. I want to see him learn. I want to be a part of that. I need to be a part. So that's a big driver in the motivation here.

Michael, forty-three years old, was diagnosed nine months before our interview. Going back a couple of years before his diagnosis, when his son was about six or seven months old, he was working for a construction company. He had been, as he put it, "relatively miserable with my job for several years." He was trying very hard to find a way out of the industry and interviewing at various other jobs he thought would be good for him. Unfortunately, he wasn't able to find that for quite some time, so he started a city job.

His son and his wife have become Michael's focus. Although he has two older daughters from a prior relationship, they live in another state, and he does not get to see them regularly. He enjoys taking his son to the zoo and going to the park down the street. He grew to enjoy his job, especially doing things for the public. It became "a matter of pride working through a city and figuring out the ins and outs of how a city runs." Also, with his daughters being much older, Michael's son was "a brand new start." Their son is his wife's only child, and Michael remarks that "they're my life, as if it started over in regard to being a dad, which I have enjoyed every bit of."

However, along with the joy and meaning in family, there is another side to the matter. For someone with cancer, having children brings an existential ache. For Linda, it is so troubling that she has wished she had not had children now that she has developed cancer. She explained,

If I had known that I was going to have this disease and be taken from them, I probably would not have had them. But I didn't know that. Now, here I am. I have to do everything that I can for them while I can.

With her children in mind, this means that she ought to do everything for their sake. With family, there is meaning.

Also, there is pain.

The magnitude of our struggle when we think of our family reflects how meaningful their existence is to us.

Service Is Purpose and Purpose Is Service

I'm a family doctor," was the first thing I would say about myself when I met people in social settings. The second thing was that I am a university professor. I took pride in serving others and found meaning in being in academia.

When I was diagnosed with cancer, one of the hardest things for me was losing the identities of doctor and teacher. Beyond not living long, what troubled me was that I wasn't sure I would be able to do what is meaningful to me while I am still alive.

At that point, I could no longer serve in both of those capacities, and that made the experience particularly hard. I took three months off from working as a doctor before returning on a part-time basis, and everyone understood. Announcing that I was diagnosed with Stage 4 lung cancer was a good enough reason for my colleagues to cover all my duties. But not being there to fulfill those duties caused a crisis in my identity.

As I grappled with how to reconstruct who I am, I thought I would want to spend the rest of my life doing what I—and only I—could do.

But this is hard to figure out.

What is it that any individual, and only that individual, does or can do? Obviously, to family and friends, the person can be valued as they are, and no one can replace them, but in other spaces, people are often thought of as interchangeable. Could there be a place for the cultivated authenticity of a person who serves and participates in the conversations, bringing what only they can bring?

My training as a doctor has given me perspectives and insight. I pursued graduate training in a master's program and then finished a PhD to learn how to understand things. But then cancer gave me perspectives I did not have before.

The illness is a real teacher. It led me down the path to my authentic self more quickly. I happen to come into contact with the experiences of other cancer patients who are, like me, grappling with similar crises, and I realized that my experience as a cancer patient is adding to what I was able to contribute before. It was almost like going to school again to learn new ways of thinking.

The experience of living with cancer was transformative.

Now, I can serve better, and I can do things for others in ways I was never able to before. To my patients, I can be the doctor who also understands their experience because he is a patient himself. I can serve communities of patients as a researcher who understands their experiences inwardly because he is also a member of and belongs in these communities.

I found purpose and authentic conversations in serving others and in being with others as they pursue what is of value to them and what is right. This is also what many of my cancer friends thought. Some found meaning in the volunteer opportunities where they came to serve other community members. Nicole puts it in a bold statement:

Purpose is a service, and service is a purpose.

For her, this is important in terms of "basic humanity." It is how she sees the world and being human. Nicole was fifty-five when we talked, and she'd had her illness for eleven months. She describes herself as a "late career academic." She had been teaching writing, literature, and film in an academic setting for nearly thirty years. Her career had been "pretty typical and involved publishing, attending conferences, and serving on and chairing committees at my institution."

She had "a very, very busy life." She would rise pretty early, about five or six in the morning, take care of some household things, and then take the dog for a walk. She lived close enough to school that she could walk or ride her bicycle to the campus. There, she would handle all her correspondence, and get ready for the several classes she usually taught every day, preparing the materials she needed and reviewing what she was teaching that day. And in between, she would meet with students and attend committee meetings. At the end of the day, she generally tried to go to the gym and exercise a little bit. Then she would go home, make some dinner, watch a bit of news, grade some papers, and "collapse around 11:00 p.m."

For Nicole, the meaning in life is simple, "If you can do something for someone else, then you should."

The desire to serve is also what made Sarah think of becoming a coach. She has seen, in her experience of health care, how professionals come to help people who are struggling, and she admires their commitment. For Sarah,

> Finding meaning was the driving force for why I've decided to go into coaching, because I felt so supported when I was sick, by not only friends and family but also the health care professionals I had along the way. I'm like, "Wow. There are a lot of people out there who could benefit from some support. What can I do? How can I help other people?" Because that's going to make me feel better, too. That's going to get me out of always thinking of me—"How can I help other people?"

She laughed as she mentioned getting out of always thinking of herself. Sarah was forty-three years old when we talked, and she'd had her cancer for nine months. Her background is in journalism and publishing. She said, "My entire career, I've been in some form of writing or research or publishing."

She had found a job as a salesperson with a self-publishing company. Authors of any genre wanting to publish their book and who were willing to invest in the publishing program would use her company. She is also a published author and thought it was a good fit. But then she was let go from her job. She found another similar job, but it paid commission only. When she was diagnosed with cancer, and after her early period of recovery, she decided not to go back to the commission-only job. She laughed as she explained to me, "Dudes, I don't have time to just keep working this job without getting paid. I need a real job."

Her dad helped her discover that she could go on disability and go back to school, and she is getting a certificate through a coaching school. When we spoke, she had just finished classes and was studying for the tests. The following month, she would be sitting for the examination and getting certified. She explained,

> I decided if I only have a couple of years left on this planet,

> I'm going to do what I want to do. I'm not going to work
> at Starbucks. Nothing against Starbucks, but I want to do
> something meaningful to me.

When we are helped, we come to realize that we, too, can help others. The act of helping and serving gives us meaning. Cancer patients also realize the struggle of the person who receives a new cancer diagnosis. They have gone through that experience themselves, and because they realize how difficult it can be, they want to make the journey more tolerable for other survivors.

This is Stephanie explaining how she finds meaning in talking to other survivors:

> When somebody is newly diagnosed, they're so scared. Being
> able to say to them, "Yup, been there, done that. I know how
> you feel. They gave me six months, but I'm in remission," I'm
> here to tell them it can be done. Because I know what that
> feels like, too, to be that new person, and wonder what's going
> to happen. And it's not that I don't wonder that, but I just keep
> fighting.

Stephanie feels she can help the person who is newly diagnosed wrap their head around the diagnosis so they can realize that it is not the end for them. She knows from her experience that there are treatments and options. She reflected on her own experience when she was diagnosed and how she started to search for any information:

> I googled everything in the beginning, and the survival rates
> aren't great, but the studies are really old, and that's one of
> the other reasons why, if I can get involved in any studies, I'd
> like to do that.

She knows from personal experience that this is scary, and if she can help others not be as scared as she was, she will do it. She understands others' suffering because she suffered, and she does not want others to suffer in the same way. Stephanie was thirty-seven when we talked, and she'd had the diagnosis for thirteen months. She explained about her life before cancer:

"It was always my dream to have my own children, to get married." She is a nurse. A year before her diagnosis, her brother, who has an intellectual disability, went into respiratory failure and was put on a ventilator. Being the nurse in the family, she had him moved to live by her in a skilled nursing facility. Her passion and dream job were in the field of intellectual disabilities, and that is what she was offered in her first job.

On a typical day, she would go out and do assessments and medical screenings to see what the patient's needs were. She also has an interest in behavioral health, and said, "If someone would be difficult psychiatrically or neurologically, I would be the one to go out to do their assessment." She also did follow-up screenings and educated facility staff about the illness processes the patient was experiencing. She noted, "If the individual wanted to learn about it, I would educate them." After cancer, Stephanie took a new job, and now she is a case manager. She works with patients who have chronic conditions, and she chooses the ones with cancer.

When we talked, she was still relatively new to the job, having been in the position for only a few months. She does not tell her patients about her diagnosis because health care professionals are advised to separate and contain their personal experiences. However, she feels differently toward those with cancer. She explained,

> I do feel a different connection with them, and I find myself probably trying to reach out to them more. When they're having a bad day, I like being able to reflect with them, just not saying, "I know what it's like because I've been there too," but just phrasing it a little bit different.

Stephanie knows that many of her patients who have other chronic conditions struggle with loss as well.

> Heart failure is a big one among our patients. I would think with any chronic condition, there's still some sense of loss because there are things that you can't do that you used to be able to.

Stephanie understands better now the experiences and struggl these patients.

You do not need to be in health care to serve. Many of the participants found meaning in returning to work, volunteering, and helping others. These not only give a sense of purpose but also put us in touch with what "normal" people do. My friends here would say,

> It is fun, and it is good.

There is also in it the human interaction with people. Service means doing work that incorporates one's talents. Whether the person is doing marketing, advertising, or any other job, it can be fun and can be meaningful when that element is included. It is also doing something that we enjoy and something that we are good at.

There is meaning in the interactions with people at work and in helping people solve problems and teaching them something. It is fun when you see that light bulb go on, and you know you've created a connection for them or an understanding.

It is just continuing to live a good, intentional life.

Part Two:

BUILDING RESILIENCE

How do people find strength?

The diagnosis of cancer and life with the illness create significant adversity. So how do people develop resilience? How do they keep going? That is what I came to explore in this part of the interviews.

People's responses varied. There were those who said that they are this certain way and always have been. They relied on themselves and took pride in being determined and strong-willed individuals. There were also those who considered the relationships in their lives to be the most important sources of their resilience. Relationships included not only family and friends but, for cancer patients, even the wider community of cancer patients. Knowing more was how some of these people felt empowered. Empowerment came through knowledge, especially knowledge about their illness, its prognosis, and the available treatment options.

For others, once again, religion arose as a source of strength. Relying on divine power was necessary for some. Not everyone, however, felt strong. Some participants felt broken inside.

I confess that I took on the endeavor of exploring how people find strength despite having many reservations about the notion of "strength." I think there is too much emphasis in our culture today on being, or at least appearing, strong.

I realize that this notion can be dangerous and burdensome. Dangerous, because it pressures people and sways them from being their authentic selves. Burdensome, because it can lay heavily on the person's conscience and demand of them to be or appear what they are not.

At the same time, the notion of strength carries social currency. It is salient in people's minds. When I asked the question, people gave replies that engaged with the topic. They even referred to having conversations with others about the issue.

The exploration is justified.

When I reconstructed the findings of my interviews here, I became convinced that the notion of resilience is just as relevant, and it is intertwined with the notion of strength. Here, what I mean by "resilience" is to be able to carry on despite a significant challenge.

Many of the survivors were resilient.

Whether the person chooses to look at the matter without being troubled by the notions of strength or resilience, I think there are lessons to be learned from the conversations I had on this topic.

Living with cancer is an experience of struggle that often shakes the person to their roots. Some come (if I allow myself to advance this plant-based metaphor) to illness with stronger and deeply grounded roots. Others grow more as they live with cancer. Still others feel as though the wind is about to carry them off the ground. We can all learn from those who are strong or resilient. In the following pages, I want to celebrate those who can teach us about resilience and real strength.

But maybe it is also OK to *not* be resilient or strong. If we accept not being strong, we open ourselves up to our vulnerability, and we become more authentic to our true selves.

Being authentic is good, too.

I Have Always Been Resilient

---

ancer affects people from all walks of life. Some of these cancer patients have dealt with adverse conditions before. They had previously been tested. Their previous experiences made them feel empowered and resilient.

When I asked James how he finds the strength, he shared a reflection about his previous hardships. People have to work to build endurance for life's struggles, he answered.

> I've always been the sort of person who adapts to and gets comfortable in the environment around me. That probably stood me in good stead with getting diagnosed.

Some people bring resilience to the experience of illness; they come with it.

Along the same lines was Amy's answer. She took pride in being determined and having carried on through difficult times. This is what Amy said:

> By nature, I'm a strong-willed person. I've always been a persistent person and kept my eye on the goal. I try to take all my life experiences, whether they're personal or career-wise, and apply it to get through the day in and day out. Whether it's how to deal with administrative staff, how to put a team together, or how to just show up as you are and let people see who you are and how you're truly feeling by being transparent. I've always, well, I shouldn't say "always"; for the majority of my adult life, I have been that way.

Amy similarly asserts that she has been a strong person most of her life.

At first, I was troubled to hear this because it appeared to me to be a claim to a strength that is not explainable. I thought of it as the same as someone saying, "I was born this way!" and that is that. But that is not really what they are saying. Being strong, in the sense of being resilient and perseverant, is an attribute of their self-identity. Being that to oneself and the world is an essential part of who the person is and something that they work to maintain. When someone asserts, "I am a strong-willed person," they mean not only that they have been that way but also that they want to continue being that way. It is, in a sense, a commitment.

The individual does not always have an answer. When I asked Katherine how she finds strength, she just laughed and said, "I do not know!" She acknowledged that other people ask her the same question. She explained,

> People ask me that. They call me strong, and I think, well, I don't know if I'm strong. I don't know if I have strength. I just keep going. I like my job, and I like the people I work with, and I like the help that I provide them, so I keep doing that. I love my family and the time with them, so I keep doing that. And there isn't much time to sit and worry, so you just keep doing what you do.

To me, it was as if she was not concerned with strength so much as with keeping going with what she does and carrying on as who she is. She also did not separate the notion of strength from who she is as a person. To be strong is not so much an external attribute but rather an existential one as being, in the sense of doing.

Katherine was not the only one troubled with how to answer this question. Donna also could not provide an answer and made similar remarks,

> I don't know. I don't know. I think that people say, "Oh, you're strong, and you're positive, and how are you so strong?" but I don't really know the answer to that. I feel like I'm just doing what I'm doing.

Some participants pointed out that although they may appear resilient to others, their adversary is not as mighty as those others may think. For example, Carol had a conversation with her therapist that changed her perspective. She explained,

> I feel like I have, through the therapist, a better understanding.

It doesn't have to be a death sentence; you can try to live your life. There is so much development and research going on right now. This is going to sound funny, but she said, "This is the best time to get cancer. Like, if you were to get cancer twenty years ago, you wouldn't be taking targeted therapy, like the one pill a day type of thing."

Here we have someone who felt broken inside but then rallied to feel she could do it and beat this disease. This sense of empowerment came after she shifted how she thought of cancer itself. In a sense, it is not death; it is just another disease. The patient does not have to surrender; they can carry on and survive. This makes the person feel stronger with regard to their condition.

Cancer is no longer a death sentence. You can still try to live life, and the challenge is not as bad as we used to think.

Family

Family provides support and confidence. In the ups and downs of the illness, having this stability gives you the strength to endure and the resilience to keep going. During the struggle, having a positive person around who provides reassurance, support, and information is essential.

Those who have children persevered because they wanted to see their children grow up. Some with children carried on also because they had no choice: their children were too young and still depended on them.

In these cases, the patient recognizes that they are loved, and if they break, others will suffer as well. They do what they can to stay around for the sake of those who love them. Some also realize that they would make others sad if they are seen as weak, and that is why they try to appear strong.

Family is important. The person with cancer appreciates them for providing the conditions that help them to carry on. Cancer shakes up a person's life, and there are ups and downs that come with it. A tight-knit family who provides stability becomes a tremendous source of support that gives you the strength you need to endure in the face of the uncertainty.

This is how Brandon described it:

> I'm very tight-knit with my family. I think it's helped me a lot, probably, having a good, stable family relationship. The relationship has been solid and stable. And it has been there both before I was diagnosed and now.

This stable ground and tight connection maintain a person's ability to carry on. Family members also provide a certainty in life that you need after your existence is shaken to the core with dread. It helps to have someone who is grounded and can laugh at the illness with you. This is what Michael had to say about it:

> My wife is so supportive and confident that when we have friends around, she likes to say that she'll be the one to kill me,

not cancer, in the end. So it helps to have her be so confident and stable.

This confidence and stability help the person. Maintaining humor also brings the person to connect with a sense of normalcy that, at times, can be threatened. We see with Michael this desire for certainty, for someone positive, for someone who can assure you that you will be all right for the time being.

Over and over, the notion of positivity and support came up. We find it also in Elizabeth's answer. It is her husband who is positive, and it is a positivity that is not based on thin air but is grounded in information he and his sister had gathered for her when Elizabeth was still too tired to even formulate a question, let alone search for the answer. She explained,

> I get strength from my husband. He's a huge source of strength for me, and from his sister, whom I would call one of my best friends. She is unbelievably positive, and she finds the good in everything and possibilities in anything. She researched the disease and treatment options before I even fully understood what was going on, when I was still in the hospital.

Having this positivity, which I interpret as confidence and optimism, is what is valued by some of these patients. It is also having reliable people around who have the agency to go beyond what is being asked of them and to seek information and help you learn more about your condition. They do this on their own for the person's sake and in the person's best interests.

Elizabeth also has another source of strength, her children.

> I get strength from my kids. I want to be around just as long as I can to see as much as I can. So for me to keep going, I get strength from watching them and looking at them, knowing that I'm their example and that I need to be the best I can be so they see that, regardless of what we are going through.

For Elizabeth, strength comes from both the desire to see her children grown and the desire to appear well to set an example for them. Seeing children grow up becomes a source of determination to carry on. You want to be around to see your children in the places you desire for them. This is what Cynthia had to say on the subject:

> I draw strength from the fact that I have a real determination to see them through to, if not adulthood, to see them through... I don't give myself deadlines because then I'd be disappointed not to make them. I dream of seeing my daughter graduate from high school. I dream of seeing where she's going to college and what she'll end up doing. So those things, that's a big strength for me. It keeps me determined to do everything I possibly can to be here for all of those things.

We do not fully understand death, and for some, living is a task, a volition. While they realize the constraints of their existence, they still give themselves license to dream and allow themselves to express their desires and their goal to be alive to see their children grow up.

This determination to carry on is not a choice for some. When children are too young, they depend on you, and you can feel you ought to carry on for that reason. This is how Katherine explains it:

> I have kids. They are young; one is only two years old. I have to look after them. I have to deal with this. I don't have much choice.

This is a commitment and a responsibility, not a preference or a desire. People do not want to live just because their dependents need them (fulfilling the needs of a child is a good example). Rather, they want to live because their loved ones want them to be in their lives. That is how Scott explained it:

> My wife wants me to hang around with her, so . . . We've known each other for a long time, since I was five years old. Our families were close, so we used to play together.

Scott is doing it for his wife, and he feels that if his wife wants him alive, he ought to stay alive. Furthermore, people want to be strong so that their family can be positive; they avoid appearing shaken so that others can maintain their composure. That is what Nancy was referring to when she said with regard to her family, "I try to be strong for them, too, because if I share my sadness, they get sad."

It is a fact that some get strength from those who support them. Others see their own sadness reflected in the eyes of those who understand and care about them. We often avoid expressing sadness so that others do not feel sad for us.

It is multilayered and complicated, for sure.

But regardless of how the family makes a person stronger, someone with cancer often feels indebted to their family. Some here thought it was because of their families that they made the right choices. Richard put it this way:

> My strength is completely dependent upon my love for my family. If I didn't have a family, then I wouldn't have much strength. I could make all the wrong choices. I could choose a negative side to things. I don't do that because they love me, and the better I am, the more they're going to appreciate that.

It is as if there is always a tension between desires and multiple other options. Richard makes his choices based on priorities related to his family. He is grateful to them for making him choose what is best for him. He feels that if he did not have his family, he would be making the wrong choices.

We are free beings, and we can be dangerous to ourselves if we choose the wrong path. But family guides us, and we can choose the right path because we love them.

Friends

The word "friends" came up often in the conversation, after "family," as a source of strength and resilience. People drew support and strength from those they connected with and who were close to them, because people appreciate feeling that they are not alone. They also appreciate those who reach out and express support and love.

Friends are especially appreciated because family is often taken as an unconditional love, while friendship is something people work on.

Cancer afflicts people individually, and many cannot help but feel alone dealing with it. They are struggling while others are carrying on with their lives. It is an isolating disease, and friends can help battle this feeling by being around and making the person feel not alone.

This is how Sandra explained it:

> I have a lot of friends who are just very supportive, and they would email me and say I'm not alone, they'll be praying for me. It just would give me comfort that I'm not alone, that people are thinking about me, and that people will help me get through it.

When friends reach out, they take the person out of their feeling of isolation. Friends are appreciated, and it is comforting to the person to know they are around.

The notion of being in others' thoughts helps as well, even when friends express their care in a language that is not precisely how the person chooses to understand the world. Michael gave an example:

> I constantly have people reaching out to me, asking how I'm doing, that I'm in their thoughts, I'm in their prayers. I'm not a spiritual person by any means, but my daughters and my friends and family who are spiritual are adding me to their prayers. I've no idea if that's going to improve my situation,

but it certainly can't hurt.

Even though he is a nonbeliever, the human connection of prayers and sending thoughts had meaning for him. He appreciated the support and kindness of the act.

I asked Stephanie to elaborate on how friends give her strength, and she explained,

> You know, even if you're having a bad day, they're still there. They'll come and do things, or if I'm up by where I used to live, I can get together with some of them.

Friends support the person's resilience by being there on those bad days. Is this not what being a friend means? They are friends because they are there in the good and bad. Our friends are those who are reliable, and reliable ones can become our friends.

The support and care granted by friends do not go unnoticed by the person with cancer, who feels grateful for the love and support given to them. It gives them resilience, strength, and love, and that is appreciated. This is how Ashley described it:

> I've got lots and lots of cards and text messages and packages in the mail. It has been great, and I've saved all those cards. And I'll go through them if I'm having a low day. I go through and reread all those, and I read those messages and think of how much it means to me to have that support. I'm aware and grateful and mindful of all the friends who have stayed with me through this and sent me good wishes and checked to see how I am and checked to see if I need anything. I appreciate that a lot, and I give a lot of thanks for that.

I could not help but think about this sentiment and how people wonder what they could do for someone with cancer and whether what they do by sending good thoughts and wishes mean anything.

Yes, those things do matter, at least to people who view the world like Ashley does and find meaning in connectedness.

Knowing More about The Disease

Knowledge about the illness makes those with cancer stronger. They become more able to hold onto positivity and optimism. They learn about treatment options and become more reassured that they will be all right. Even those who deal with recurrence can still feel reassured, because they know more and can hold on to hope. As patients realize the empowerment that comes with knowing, they want to know more so they can make the best decisions.

People often speak about certainty, or call it positivity. It is at the center of what gives people more peace of mind and a better ability to look forward. It is a framework through which to look at the matter, and some argue that it can be a choice.

There is what I would call a "blind positivity," which a cancer patient often does not buy. This is reassurance that is not based on truth. There is also a genuine positivity that comes when optimism is based on a fact that gives grounds for hope.

Knowing about the illness provides better conditions for the person to find a grasp on positivity. Mary referred to this type of positivity:

> I'm finally to the point where I feel like I'm going to live awhile and that when something does happen, like the disease progressing, I know there's another medication that I can take, and it is going to take care of that.

Mary's disease did progress and, when we talked, she was dealing with a recurrence. Her husband was devastated, but she held strong to a positivity anchored in knowledge and hope.

> You know, it's just the next step in my journey where we're going to get out a better medicine. This one is going to do the job, and I feel at peace now.

What helps to give her strength is knowing that there are other treatment options. She is certain, and that is because of what she knows. There are newer treatments, and that is a fact. So her strength comes with her certainty in knowing that fact. She can now assert, without a doubt, that she will be all right because if this medicine fails, there will be another one.

This knowledge gives her strength.

Not having this certainty leaves room for fear. David reflected on this, saying that in the beginning, "there was a fear of what the next step would be." He explained that he had gotten better at dealing with it. A turning point was his visit to the oncologist, who then talked to him about other options for treatment. The oncologist spoke about immunotherapy that he could do afterward. He shared that "when I left that visit, I was finally optimistic. I just came home like I was walking on air."

What helps David stay strong is knowing that there are options. After talking to his oncologist, he felt reassured again, and now he can have less fear and more peace. There are treatment options, and he is confident of that. This is positivity.

Learning about the disease has helps the person and gives strength even in face of uncertainty. Here, Susan said, "Just the knowledge, because I am a nurse" was a help. Susan is also active in the online group. She explains, "I try to learn as much as I can and research it and look at trials."

It also reassures her to learn about experts in the world of oncology who are available and doing work on her mutation. People with similar experiences helped, she explains, "people will give me an answer, and so that group has been very instrumental also."

Other participants find the information useful for dealing with their condition. Ashley explained,

> I haven't gone through the files yet because I'm pretty new
> to the group, but I know that there's a lot of information and
> research in the file and examples. When they post something
> new, I try to do some research of my own on it and find
> out what does that mean, what's that about? How does that
> apply to me? I take notes so that I can discuss it with my son,
> who's been very active in researching all these topics and
> getting answers. So the medical research is good to have but it

basically, for me it's a tool to know what to ask my oncologist about if there's a question or something that I want to have answered. It gives me a format for it.

She tries to research and find information and answers. And there is a lot of information out there. Her family is also active in researching. Ashley wants to have answers because they empower her in face of her disease.

Learning from the community was that which gave strength for others. Cynthia remarked,

> It's like the more involved and educated I become and the more connections that I make in that community, the more hopeful I feel and the more hopeful I feel for the patients who are going to come after me.

Being educated empowered Ashley, Cynthia, and those like them. Cynthia realizes that learning is an essential way to deal with the disease, and she feels hopeful for herself and other cancer community members when she learns.

Some participants took it upon themselves to be able to converse knowledgeably with their doctors. They don't want to just let others decide for them. Andrew reflected on this viewpoint:

> So, I often do my own research, but it's research that's real research. I'm not looking at secondhand sources. I was looking for a specific study and signed up for the *New England Journal of Medicine* so that I could read this whole article, and I learned a bunch of stuff that was very useful to me. I believe if I'm going to do what I promised my kids to do, which was to shoot for any reasonable open window, I have to be able to converse about the topic. I can't understand at the level the doctors do, but I at least need to understand what's happening to me and be able to be a critical thinker in the decision-making rather than just saying, "OK, that's the drug you recommend? Let me go for it."

Andrew looks up resources, including original research studies and original articles. He realizes that it is OK to not understand at the doctor's level, but for himself, he wants to be able to converse with doctors. For Andrew, the patient should not just follow recommendations without critically thinking about them. Andrew promised his kids to shoot for every possibility, and that is why it is essential to him to have the capacity to dialogue about these possibilities.

Another person who asserted that knowing more provides better conditions for dealing with the disease was Amy. She has a recurrence, but she is "staying positive." She explained that she and her family are doing a lot of research, and they have appointments for further studies. She is also going to a major cancer center to meet a specialist in her mutation (EGFR). But it is still devastating. She explained,

> I felt like I was getting back on my feet. I was doing better, and then I got cut down at the knees. It's now . . . everything is up in the air, and it's similar to the feeling of the initial diagnosis.

Amy shared that when she sits still and thinks about it, she cries.

It is tough to be thrown back to the starting point of suffering you thought you had left behind.

But Amy is not sitting and waiting for the fate; she is trying to learn more so she can make more educated decisions. Amy explained this:

> Currently, most of my time has been spent reading about my cancer, reading about research, speaking, setting up appointments, getting my team to give me feedback on different tests and what they think the next plan of action should be so I can make educated decisions.

Amy was devastated by her recurrence, but she is holding strong. While she is thrown back to the place where she is dealing again with uncertainty, Amy is not the same person. She explained,

> The difference is that now I have so much more knowledge. I have so many more connections. I have so much more support.

I know that there are other clinical trials out there that could help me and will help my fellow lung buddies, and in that, I stay strong from the faith, from hope, from persistence.

She has more knowledge, and she has more support. She knows more, she has more connections, and she knows that both her knowledge and her relationships will help her. So she is not in the same place.

Yes, the existential threat is still looming.

But she is not the same person, and she knows that.

Religion

Religion can not only give meaning but can also provide strength and support resilience. Some people resumed a connection with their faith after their diagnosis, while others have always had their faith at the center of their life. The rituals help some stay strong. Others are supported by the frame of reference that explains life and gives an answer about what will happen afterward. Religion, however, is not the answer for everyone.

Some people returned to church after they became ill. This is what Jessica answered when I asked about how she gets strength:

> We did go back to church; we hadn't been for years. We are not super involved, just on Sunday.

In returning to church, there is a community found and a sense of belonging.

Others, like Richard, have had spirituality as a constant quest.

> In terms of my spirituality, God, I never put it down. All the questions and curiosity have been piqued in terms of looking for signs; "Am I going to be OK in the afterlife?" So that's a constant quest.

In that constant quest is a connection to something beyond, and there is empowerment.

Knowing what will happen after death is particularly important here. That is what Rebecca explained when I asked about what helped her get strength:

> First of all, my faith. My prayer life might help in keeping my thought process in knowing that if I were to die, I'd be OK. I feel that because of that, I've been more effective in my life. Having that peace helps me and gives me inspiration that I can keep doing things and making things better for people around me. So, I think that's what gives me strength; it is knowing I'm

effective and I'm being intentional about what I'm doing. I'm
not just sitting back and letting life rant at me.

Faith gives her strength, and it is not in isolation from living life day-to-day. She takes pride in being intentional and effective, and faith gives her the strength to do that rather than just sitting back and letting life take over.

Some also find strength in looking for signs. Sandra shared that she watches for signs so she can know that God will be with her. She gave me some examples of the signs she looks for:

> We were going to the oncologist's office, and we took a wrong
> turn and ended up in the parking lot of a Lutheran church.
> I'm Lutheran, and so I told my husband, maybe that's a sign.

They started going to the same church after that. Going to church was something she had not done for many years. She also shared another example:

> I was having a rough time, and the pastor, who was a high
> school classmate, sent me a little text, and it had some scripture,
> Psalm 23. It was very comforting. Then, that next Sunday
> was the first Sunday when we were going to that church, and
> we got there and heard the scripture was Psalm 23, the same
> scripture.

Psalm 23 reads, "Even though I walk through the darkest valley, I will fear no evil, for you are with me; your rod and your staff, they comfort me."

The signs give her strength.

While some are observant to the meaning and signs of their faith, other participants take a more practical approach and emphasize what the rituals do for them. Stephanie said,

> My religion helps as a stress release, you know, a place to go to
> get out of your head again. Just to have that quiet time.

Praying helps with their stress. And religion helps them get out of their own heads and let go of the stress.

However, religion is not the answer for everyone. As a matter of fact, for some, it was a frustration that all conversations in their smaller community were religiously focused. While they desired human connection, religion was a deterrent in relationships with others. Lisa explained it this way:

> I'm not much of a just-sit-around-and-do-nothing type of person, yet we don't know a lot of people here yet. So, we don't have a big social life, because it's hard meeting people because it's always going to come back to Jesus. It's just my hot button.

Lisa moved to a smaller town, and she is struggling to find community. She does not have school-aged children so that she would meet other parents, and she does not belong to the church. She explained further,

> Every support group I've ever tried to look at or go to, it always comes back to Jesus, and I can't do that. That's not who I am.

It troubled her once when she was in the hospital and the staff were saying prayers before a procedure. One person explained that they were praying for her and were going to take care of her. She shared her thoughts on this:

> I'm thinking, like, "OK, what movie am I in?" I respect everybody's religious views, but I also want to be able to not have them tied to care. I mean, I have a hard time if anybody in the medical situation says, "We're going to pray about it." No!

Lisa does not want to offend anyone, but *she* gets offended. She explained,

> It offends me for people to think that their prayers have something to do with the care that I deserve as a patient . . . I know so many people when they answer your question, "I find that strength with my faith," and I can't answer that question that way.

Faith gives strength to some people.

But not all people.

No Strength

A t times, we cannot be strong. At times, we do not want to be strong. And it is OK to let go.

Strength is not something people can always access. Lisa would say that it should be OK to not have strength at times. She has always considered herself a "really strong person," but there are times when she does not want to be strong anymore. Those are the times when the strong sense of self-worth becomes a burden, when the person wishes to let go.

Lisa confessed how hard it is to be the one who holds it together all the time. At times, she wants to let go and not keep it together anymore. She shared about the times when that has happened:

> One time, when I was in the hospital, I had a total breakdown because I was missing my dog so badly.

She has a two hundred and forty pound Mastiff, and all she wanted to do "was to hold and see the dog." As Lisa was sharing this moment, she realized that she was sharing vulnerability, so she explained,

> I mean, everybody has those moments. I just started crying. I just started crying. It had been a particularly difficult day in the hospital. All of a sudden, I didn't want to be there. I didn't care. I didn't care if I was going to—I didn't care what the consequences were for a moment or two; I just wanted to be out of there.

That was a breaking point for Lisa. Sometimes the person needs to let go. We all have our breaking point. At times, strength is just not attainable.

Linda spoke about that:

> Sometimes, I don't feel I have strength. Some days, I feel broken. I feel I can't do it for another day. I remember thinking to myself one time, maybe shouting it out loud when I was newly diagnosed, and I was running. I was out for a run. "I cannot do it!"

She has times when she doesn't feel strong and only feels broken inside. Who doesn't have that? However, when the person surrenders to those states, they sometimes bounce back immediately. This is the bottom that we can hit and then bounce back off of.

Linda added,

> But then I look at those girls and my husband. I think about wanting to be there for them. I was telling myself, "This is the best you're gonna feel for the rest of your life. So either you have to just shut up and do it, or you can keep going downhill." That was a turning point for me. I thought to myself, "OK. Well, right now, this is the best I'm going to feel for the rest of my life. And so I might as well enjoy it." It sucks that this is where it is, but I can either sit there and think how much it sucks or get up and live. I think I would rather get up and live.

Linda does not always have the strength to carry on. But she does have this feeling that motivates her and gets her out of bed every morning. To her, it sucked, and that is not how she would have designed her life. However, she *chooses* to get up and live.

She wants to carry on.

How Do I Find Strength?

This question is not easy, and I have to confess, now that I am putting myself in place to answer, that I get strength not from one but rather from many things.

As I write these words, I feel some guilt about the research participants because I wish I could have given everyone the same space to say what they want as I have, and then I could put it all together in a meaningful way.

When I reflect now on finding strength and resilience, of course, I am at a vantage point to know myself because I can sit and think about it. I can also take the time to write and edit. But most importantly, my vantage point has to do with writing this after I learned from all the other participants how *they* find strength.

I am over the guilt and would rather live with no regret, and I am authoring this book, so why not give myself a few extra pages? Plus, if I open myself to others, maybe they can also think again and share more. Wouldn't it be wonderful if everyone opened their souls and shared with everyone else?

That is the task I have set for myself here. I will share a few reflections about how I found strength and built resilience.

My Family

I am fortunate to be the youngest of nine siblings, to have their love and caring along with the love and caring of my dad. They do not live close to me, but they have always been very supportive.

Indeed, I did not want them to visit as much when I became ill. I tried to carry on with my life. But I knew they were there for me. I knew that I have unconditional love and support. I also wanted to be resilient for them so that they could maintain resilience. But I also wanted to be vulnerable, open, and authentic with them so they could be all of that with me as well, and so they can better deal with my struggle and their struggle.

My family does not always say what I think is the right thing. But they are not shy about calling me out on my bullshit. They always said that I could do more, whether that was staying fit and exercising or enjoying life or working harder.

They held me accountable for maintaining a better version of myself, and for that, I thank them.

Crystal

Crystal is my fiancée and my lover. I have always said that she outsmarts me and out-compassions me. I mean it.

She is a pediatrician who takes care of kids from immigrant and refugee families. She complains about the system because she wants her children to have better health care, the health care they deserve.

She has many more stamps in her passport than I do, and she is fluent about good food.

Crystal knows how to listen and not judge. She cares, and she taught me to open my soul to her and to be vulnerable because she cares.

And when I grow distant as I sink into the pain and fear, we always find time to break the coldness with tears and snuggles.

Leonardo

Leonardo, or Leo, is my German Shepherd. Leo knows me, and he is my real friend. I adopted him when he was eight weeks old, at a time when I thought love was impossible. I wanted the unconditional acceptance that I felt only a dog would give. And he did.

Leo knows how to look into my eyes and see through me. He knows how to put his paw in my hand as we commit to an eternal trust (or when he is hungry).

I was once worried that I might outlive him, and it ached me to think that he would only live for a little over ten years. I decided to get a puppy once Leo gets old so the puppy and I can console each other when Leo passes away.

When I developed cancer and realized that he might outlive me, it became urgent to me to find him a home where he is loved, in case I could not take care of him anymore. And I did find him a second home.

But then I found us Crystal and Crystal's dog, Sammy. Sammy and Leo are more of platonic friends, and they have their debates. If I were to guess, I would say they debate which treats taste better.

Leo will be all right, and I am OK because I have Leo.

Reading and Writing

I read philosophy and, with practice, have developed the capacity to deal with complex ideas. I also write, and that has become one way of making sense of my struggle. Philosophy deals with the abstract but also provides frameworks you can bring to daily experiences. And writing gives you the freedom to reconstruct meaning and develop language to comprehend.

I was able to develop a language that made sense of my struggle. I developed tools that then reshaped who I was. My work on these tools is not dissimilar to a statue at the Seattle Art Museum, where the sculpture sculpted the wooden tools that carved them!

We recreate ourselves when we rewrite our words.

With learning, especially philosophy, we develop our tools to recreate ourselves.

My Values and Commitments

When I became ill, it was urgent for me to be authentic to myself. At the same time, it was essential that I not have regrets in the sense that I do not die with a feeling that I have wronged someone else. This truthfulness to myself and, at the same time, care for what others think has become the grounds for how I think about what is good and what is right.

Every person matters, and they matter equally.

To do what is right for others became essential to me because if I were to focus only on what is relevant to me, I would be vain and die in my own vanity. I did not want that. I wanted this to be a better place after me, in the sense of a more just place.

Also, as I was battling my fear of death, lesser threats became trivial. I had not been shy about speaking truth before, but with my illness, I cultivated an empowered voice. I took a stance on things and spoke truth to power. At times, I channeled my anger toward what is not right, especially when humans treat others as less than themselves.

Because I would not be the person who sits quietly, I made commitments and announced positions on issues that matter.

And my connection to these higher values and positions has kept me standing.

My Identity

The fear of death and the formative experiences I had in confronting that have allowed me the chance to cultivate my identity and positions.

This identity came with the expectation of carrying on. I had things to do and work to achieve. That was the person I wanted to be, and that is how I wanted to be known. I had no time to lick my wounds or to wallow in self-pity.

I aspired to write my narrative and to maintain it. I wanted to be the main author of my narrative and did not want my story to be told in a way other than I would tell it.

That is not about appearances; it's about genuinely being. It is about truthfulness.

This desire to maintain my authentic identity became a force to not perform but rather to pull me up when, at times, the illness beats me down.

My Previous Experiences

I came to the experience of illness with strength.

I am an immigrant, and being an immigrant gave me resilience and stability. I had no choice but to have that resilience and perseverance. My country, Syria, is burning, and there is no going back.

Being from Syria also left me with guilt and a sense of duty. I survived, while many people did not. I must therefore do something useful with my life.

Before my illness, I was a doctor. It takes rigorous training and hard work to become a doctor. The training is not just in skills but includes, more importantly, a training of character.

I was also a researcher. I learned how to think methodically, and when I became ill, I did not leave that to the side. Rather, I used it. I did not fall off into just accepting odd answers but was able to hold on to what is fact and what is right.

I was also a teacher. I have learned to be an example, and when I became ill, I decided to continue being an example. I thought that if I am going to die, the last thing I would teach others is how to do it well.

Running Out of Time

The last thing I would reflect on here is my perception that I was running out of time. That was also a source of endurance. I had to work twice as fast as I would have had I not developed cancer, and I had to work twice as hard.

True, I was tired, and true, I was weak. My days became shorter. I lost a few hours every day because my body's demand for rest increased.

Still, I told myself that I should take the opportunity while I am here, and I need to do what I need to do. The perception of having no time in hand helped me focus. It also helped me leverage my powers and put them to good use.

With taking notes, I was not always strong. I had times when I thought this living is unbearable, and I had times when I felt broken inside. I also had times when I wanted to stop this striving.

I hit deep bottoms.

But because I was there, I am stronger now.

Part Three:

HEALTH ACTIONS

I was curious to learn what people do in the broader area of health.

I asked the question in this simple way: "What are you doing in the areas of health and well-being?" I often followed with a clarification such as "What are you doing to get and stay healthy?"

To reconstruct this part of the conversation, I have divided this section into the topics of diet, exercise, complementary and alternative medicine (CAM), and targeted chemotherapy. In each subject, I explore what people are doing or not doing and why they are doing or not doing a specific thing.

I also invited people to reflect on their experiences and share what they perceive is working or not working. I included this exploration in the book because I thought patients might want to know and learn about others' experiences. Health care providers may also want to know about patients' thought processes.

People with advanced cancer have an existential threat. With this threat comes, for some, the desire to do all that is possible to abate the danger. That is understandable. Cancer also leaves many scars, and its treatment has many complications. People want to live a more tolerable life and one of better quality.

As I included a diversity of practices, I wanted to never judge any person for whatever they do. I hoped to provide some insight from different people's experiences. I also wanted to call attention to positions that might be extreme in one direction or the other. Ultimately, I wanted to shed light on the space where someone can enact their agency to do a little more if they desire to and can. The goal may not necessarily be curing the illness but rather to live in the way they want to live.

So, this book is not about what a person should do to live better with cancer. The book is only about what some people with cancer are doing. If you want to know what you could or should do in terms of your health, speak to your doctor. You can also do your own research using trusted, evidence-based health resources.

I share remarks on what I do in the areas of health and well-being. And

I recount how I became ill. In confessing how I struggled to make sense of my illness, I hope to give people a language to deal with that question when it arises for them. I also hope to call out the prejudice against people who smoked and then developed lung cancer. While it is good to do healthy things, those choices, in the end, mostly have to do with the individual's values and preferences. It is not another person's business, including doctors, to judge or have a prejudice against the individual for their health choices.

We can do better in that area.

Diet

We all have to eat. One way or another, we make choices about our diet. While some may have paid more attention to food than others, developing cancer made most of these patients at least think about their options.

Some chose to not make changes, for varying reasons. Others decided to eat differently, and the changes varied between focusing on specific options to eliminating other components of their diet.

Those who chose to change their diets did so for a number of different reasons.

In the following pages, I will present the diversity of people's options. When I dialogued with the participants, it was harder at times to put aside my position as a doctor. When people came to me with this or that choice, I often had comments or suggestions to make. I am also personally faced with the same existential question, and I have my positions on this matter. I have also made choices related to what I eat.

What is more important to me here, however, is not to speak like the doctor or attempt to support or refute any particular choice with evidence. What is essential is not to reflect on my decision, either—I will do that at the end of the section, and I have already presented my general framework in the previous pages so do not find a need to go into specifics. I mostly want to leave the space for the participants to share their thinking and for readers to come with an open mind to understand.

I also want to provide the breadth of choices to invoke conversation and invite more inquiry.

I Choose Not to Change My Diet

Some participants did not change their diet. This choice was not because they are oblivious to the matter. One can see from the depth of reflection that they have thought about nutrition and considered the issue.

Most participants who chose not to change their diet made a deliberate and thoughtful decision.

For some, it was because they had already made changes before the illness. So there was nothing to change to bring them closer to their conception of what is healthy. For others who chose not to change their diet, it was because they were not convinced that making changes to their diet would help them in their urgent struggle. For them, the evidence is judged as limited at best. Others experienced side effects from their treatments that made them not tolerate or enjoy food. For them, any eating was good, so it didn't matter what they ate as long as they ate.

Finally, the last group I give voice to here felt that changing their diet was not worth the effort since they have advanced disease. They would rather spend their energy on enjoying life and all it has to offer, including good food.

I have already been eating healthily

As already noted, some participants had already been paying attention to their diet before the illness, and they made no changes after diagnosis. Richard is one of them, and his remarks sum it up well: "My diet didn't really change. I'd always been very conscientious about what I ate and aware of what I ate." So for him, there was no other change to make.

Similar to this position was that of Samantha, who also made no changes. She explained,

> I've always eaten good food for my diet. I just don't really eat much meat, and I mostly eat a healthy vegetarian diet. I eat other things like eggs and cheese and stuff, too. I'm not vegetarian, but I eat a lot of vegetables and grains, and I don't eat gluten. I stopped eating wheat about five years ago because I had a lot of GI upset, and it's helped to get rid of the gluten.

She described her diet as good to start with, and she did not have to make a change. Samantha's changes had been made for other health reasons long before her cancer diagnosis.

Participants' food choices were not determined only by their views of what is healthy. They are often constrained by their life's context. While someone may try to make mindful choices, they do not live in a vacuum, and their preferences cannot be steered to a drastically different course without considering others. Linda explained this circumstance:

> Honestly, I don't live differently now than I did before. I had to focus on healthy eating and healthy living. I feel all the things that I think would be good for me to do for cancer, I was doing before I was diagnosed. So it doesn't feel I'm doing those things because I have cancer. I try to have healthy eating. I'm not very rigid. I'm not over the top about it, but I've always tried to focus on healthy eating. Fruits and vegetables. I've always cooked with my kids, and we juice. We've been juicing for a long time. It's part of our day. On the weekend, I prep a lot of food for the week so that we can eat healthy when we're running around like crazy. Things like that. So eating, I've gone back and forth. I tried to do a vegan diet, but it just doesn't work when you're feeding three little kids. We try to have vegan dinners all through the week, but then on the weekends, we are a little bit less rigid. We'll have whatever it is that they want to have. We've tried different ways of making healthy eating just the expectation while also being flexible.

For these people, the question of living healthy is salient from before. And with children, one has to make choices and allow for flexibility.

I Am Not Convinced That Changing My Diet Would Do Much

Some participants didn't believe that changing their diet was going to provide a cure or make a significant impact on their outcome as cancer patients. They generally made this decision after careful investigation. Emily spoke about what she had examined:

> I looked into the diet. I looked into cancer and sugar, and that didn't seem conclusive. I asked my oncologist about it, and I have a friend who's a lymphoma researcher, and she said

cancers could metabolize whenever it can metabolize; you have to feed yourself. So I try not to make a major change.

Emily made her decision after thoughtful consideration and inquiry. Other participants were skeptical of the reasoning and effectiveness around particular dietary recommendations. Among these was Melissa, who is a nephrologist. Melissa is versed with evidence-based practice and knows how the body works. She also knows what interventions are based on facts and which ones are based on myth.

> I've got Stage 4 lung cancer. I'm not going to be drinking green shakes that taste bad. It's just not my style. That doesn't mean I'll go crazy; I like to live normally. I don't believe in any of the crazy diet stuff. You have to realize I'm a nephrologist; I don't believe in alkaline diets and all this other nonsense, because it *is* nonsense if you know physiology.

She called out the many beliefs that are not supported by objective evidence. She recognizes that people eat or drink this or that because of personal choice. Green juices were not her preference. She was clear, however, that if someone believes they will change their body's pH by drinking this or something else, then they are sailing on the wrong path.

Even without a medical degree, Larry was not convinced that his diet could change the course of his illness. He explained,

> I've probably done no diet changes. My wife tries to give me good food. But I've come across different recommendations in forums, and I understand some people feel very strongly about certain things. I think because of my wife's medical training, we said that eating well is a good thing, but it's not a cure. I don't understand the biology, the mechanics of how eating a lot of oil or something would cure me. I don't think there's research that would support that.

For them, eating well is no cure, and although they know that eating well is a good thing, they eat what they want.

If My Time Is Limited, I Want to Enjoy Different Food Choices

Some participants had the sentiment that if time on earth is constrained, why should you bother with too many restraints? Donna spoke from this mind-set:

> Quite honestly, if I am going to be dying soon, I don't want to spend my life worrying about having to eat only meat or whatever the keto diet is. It sounds terrible. So, I want to live my life normal.

For them, people who are possibly dying should not worry about what to eat and not eat. Cancer patients will get all kinds of recommendations, but they become irrelevant to someone who wants to live in the time they have left. Similarly, Mary explained,

> When I was first diagnosed, you'd get all these suggestions, "Oh, you need to be taking this. You need to be eating these kinds of food." Someone recommended a raw diet once. At this point in my life, I am eating, and I am drinking what I want and when I want, but in moderation.

People make all kinds of suggestions about diet. For some, like Mary, doing things in moderation is what is right. That was also Jessica's position. However, she experienced some of the consequences that can come from letting yourself have whatever you want:

> We all kind of thought, hey, my time is limited, you might as well enjoy life. I quit smoking, and I quit drinking. So the only other thing I guess I was replacing it with is eating whatever I wanted to eat. Now I'm still alive, a year and a half later. I'm probably going to be alive for a long time, so now I can't eat what I want to eat.

Mary shared that her next goal is to get serious about her diet so she can do what she wants to do.

> So it's time to straighten up and do something about it, and

I'm at that point right now that if I die a year from now, I still need to straighten up and do something about my exercise and my diet.

The wonderful surprise that they are still alive can make these patients want to develop healthier habits again so they can endure living without the consequences of extra weight and an unhealthy diet.

I Do Not Have Much Choice With My Diet

Some participants felt they didn't have much choice when it came to diet, and they wanted to eat anything that they could. Ashley is one of these people.

Going to the hospital, I wasn't able to eat. They were really harping on me about eating proteins, and I had been a vegan for quite some time, and I just had to allow myself to eat whatever I could swallow and keep down.

Not everyone had a choice, and at times when it is hard to keep anything down, they are OK with eating whatever they can.

Other participants who did not have much choice to make included Cynthia:

I started my treatment on chemotherapy, which has a lot of dietary issues related to it because there are foods that suddenly no longer agree with you. For me, I struggled for months with the fact that my taste buds had changed, and things that I had loved didn't taste good to me anymore. So I don't follow any special diet.

After her treatment, not all food tasted good to Cynthia anymore, so eating whatever was out of necessity rather than choice. However, when nothing tastes good, some people still chose healthier options. Here is what Rebecca had to say about this:

When I went through the chemo, I was pretty miserable, and

I've always struggled with weight. So my husband would say, "What do you want to eat?" And I'd say, "Nothing sounds good; just make something healthy because I don't care what it tastes like and it's good for my body."

Later on, Rebecca started feeling better. As part of her rehab, she took classes and learned more about how to incorporate vegetables in her diet.

Now, when I'm hungry, I tell myself, "Well, my body needs more of that protein and vegetables." I need it balanced with everything and the more I eat like that, the better I feel.

There are things the person desires, and there are things that are good for the body. Healthy is at least good for the body.

I Choose to Eat a Different Diet

Some participants made changes to their diet, and those who did so made all kinds of changes. Adding this or that food element was the choice of some, while others eliminated specific diet components. People made these changes for all sorts of reasons. Some wanted to put their bodies in the best position to deal with the illness, while others wanted to fight cancer with diet. There was, however, no consensus on whether diet choices would make a difference.

Types of diet changes

These changes ranged from eliminating sugar or animal products to increasing specific items like fruits or vegetables or avoiding foods that are processed or that had hormones added. Below, I address some of the specific categories of foods that were sometimes the target of the changes and the types of changes that were made within those categories.

Adding vegetables and fruits

For some participants, eating healthy meant more green things, including smoothies. Nancy explained it:

> My diet, I try hard to eat very healthy and do the green
> smoothies. It gives me more energy when I eat well. When I
> do the greens smoothies, it makes me feel better.

They want to eat what can be described as healthy, and that is important for them.

Another participant, Donna, added a few plant-based items. Because she takes a medicine that requires fat for absorption, she is mindful of that as well. She explains,

> I try to eat yogurt with some berries. I know the berries are
> good for me, but I have changed from nonfat yogurt to whole
> milk yogurt so that it has a little bit more fat in it. In the
> evening, I take my medication either with some almonds or
> with like a sample of peanut butter, too.

Another person who reduced meat in her diet is Nicole. She explained, "We focus a lot on vegetables and whole grain pasta, rice, quinoa, couscous." For Nicole, this food actually tastes better, but she has also become "more vigilant about it now having had cancer." She is interested in the topic and has read "a couple of cancer cookbooks" people gave her. To Nicole, it all "makes sense."

Eliminating meat and other animal products

Some people removed meat. Justin is one who made similar changes and adopted a vegan diet. He said,

> Yes, a diet change is one of the biggest things I've done. I used
> to eat meat, and the closest thing to meat I'll eat now is eggs,
> but that was a big change for me. Juicing is a big change where
> I do drink a lot of juices.

So Justin went vegan and drank more juice. Some other participants went vegan after reading a book on health. Elizabeth explained her choice to do so:

So I went vegan when I got diagnosed. I read a book about that. The author wrote all this stuff about how not to die. I know a lot of Western medicine doctors think it's a bunch of crap, but I was always using a healthy diet anyway. I also wanted to cut out the dairy, and I wanted to cut out meat.

They learned it from a book. Like many people, Elizabeth does things even though her doctors may not find them useful. It was humbling to me as a doctor to hear that, and it was a privilege. It is as if she is saying, "I know doctors don't think it's useful, but that doesn't matter." However, I couldn't help but wonder if there is not a loss when the authority of medicine is questioned in this way. Still, I put my concerns aside.

What matters is that people make choices, and they do so for different reasons.

Eliminating sugar

Some participants adopted a no-sugar diet, or what is called the ketogenic diet. Debora explained it:

On my diet, I try very low glycemic foods. I've read that cancer feeds on sugar. Cancer is a metabolic process; it's not just genetic. If you think of a PET scan and the cancer uptakes, cancer cells take up the sugar much quicker than the other cells, and that's why they light up.

She supports her practice by a belief in theory and by an analogy.

Another participant, John, also avoided sugar and adopted a ketogenic diet.

I adopted a ketogenic diet just because I kept reading that reducing cancer has to do with glucose metabolism. Cancer cells rely on glucose in the bloodstream to grow and proliferate. So, it made sense to me that reducing blood glucose levels would make my body less fertile for cancer to spread and grow. It also reduces inflammation. So, I adopted a diet about six months ago, and I've been following it ever since.

For John, this is a plausible mechanism to help with cancer.

Eating organic and avoiding GMO

Eating organic and avoiding additives became essential to some. Here is what Stephanie had to say on this type of diet:

> I eat pretty much all organic, non-GMO. That is what was recommended. I've gone to two nutritionists, and also my neurologist had given me some tips as well. As far as with the organic—not to be eating processed type foods or anything that has been injected with antibiotics—it is just more natural.

For her, eating processed foods with antibiotics is not good; instead, eating natural food is healthy. Stephanie wants to eat the healthiest diet possible. Some also eat organic and fresh food because they are available and easily accessible. Nicole reflected that she is lucky to have those options available to them. She was aware of this:

> I'm fortunate; I live in a neighborhood where I have good access to clean food. I know not everybody does, but I have access to it here, and it's also affordable. We have farmer's markets; we have a grocery that sells organic products at pretty reasonable prices. Because of that, I have more access to that kind of food, so why not take advantage of it?

Nicole's mom was a science teacher, and she grew up on a farm. The family also grew up eating a lot of fresh vegetables, so this probably influenced Nicole's choices to some extent.

Making multiple changes

Many of the participants didn't make only one of the changes I've discussed but instead made a few of them at the same time. The changes were often linked to an understanding of what a healthy diet meant to them, and that was usually multiple things. James explained,

> I made a really big change to my diet. I greatly reduced my sugar intake and greatly increased my fruit and vegetable intake. I ate a lot more healthily. I've kept on with that, and I've probably improved that diet change further. Now, I'm drinking a lot of filtered water. I'm not a fanatic about it but pretty conscientious about it.

He made a change to his diet by reducing sugar. He also began consuming more fruits and vegetables and reducing intake of processed goods with chemical additives to eat what he considers to be a healthy diet.

Some participants made multiple changes but still insisted on continuity with a previous lifestyle and enjoying good food. Donna had this viewpoint:

> I try to add more healthy things to my diet rather than changing things dramatically. I'm getting more dairy to get my calcium. I know that since I have metastasis in my bones, I'm worried about breaks. I think that adding some fruit to breakfast every day is a good idea for some antioxidants. For lunch, I'll have salad in general, trying to get some greens. For dinner, I go out to dinner a lot, so there is bad food there, and I might have dessert.

Donna clarified that bad food meant "delicious food" and added,

> I don't want to change my life dramatically because I want to be able to enjoy it as well, and nobody has given me concrete evidence that changing my diet completely would help cancer in any way. So, I live a normal lifestyle that way.

She recognizes that there is no good evidence to support the notion that any of these dramatic changes helps. Therefore, she wants to maintain some semblance of a normal lifestyle and enjoy life while also being healthy.

Reasons for the diet change

Some participants offered their reasons for making these changes. Participants with this stance wanted to do everything possible to put themselves in the best position of health as they deal with cancer. Some sought recommendations from their doctors, while others consulted books, magazines, or journals or got advice from people.

When confronted with cancer, some people want to do all they can to optimize their chances. These participants tried to do that with guidance from the experiences of experts and other people. Sarah explained this choice:

> One of the first things I did is after I found out about the support group is I started reaching out to people because I'm like, "OK, they gave me three months to live." And then they said, "Wait, you might have a year. We don't know." And I'm like, "What?" So OK, I want to do everything that I can do to get better. I reached out to people in the online support group, and I asked them, "What are you eating? What are you doing? What diet are you on?"

She wanted to do all that is within their means to optimize her chances. But when participants asked for suggestions or advice, people made all kinds of recommendations, so some tried different things to be in the best position possible. Rebecca reflected,

> I've seen on a lot of posts in forums recommending eating organic. Also, some people say, "Oh, just eat what you want." Other people say, "Make this change or that." Certain people don't eat sugar. Everybody does their own thing. I just felt that, for me, the healthiest thing I could do is what I want to do because I'm a fighter, and I want to beat this.

She explained further about doing the healthiest things:

> The healthier my body is, the better it can fight off anything that might arrive. If cancer would start to grow, I want my

body to be strong, and I want my body to have the right nutrients to be able to help fight it off. That's why I feel it's my time that I could do something to help my body fight.

Rebecca wants to help her body fight cancer by making healthy choices. However, the diversity of concrete recommendations may reflect the lack of evidence for any specific one. Maybe that is why most medical doctors would not make any one specific recommendation other than eating a healthy diet in the broader sense of the word. Still, some doctors may address the matter in more depth than others.

James recounted the conversations he'd had with his oncologist and other doctors:

My oncologist was probably very different than most oncologists. She's a DO as opposed to an MD. She has got an attitude that's more open to other therapy as well as Western medicine. Very early on, she referred me to naturopathic care. The naturopath reinforced all the changes that I was making with diet and exercise.

Seeing the naturopath was helpful, and they agreed on the common sense diet changes.

At times, when their doctors made recommendations to avoid strict dietary regimens, some participants went against the recommendations. The person does what she wants, even if the oncologist recommends the opposite. Here again is Elizabeth, talking about her choice to be vegan:

My oncologist is very against me being vegan. She was from the beginning. I didn't really care, and so I did it anyway.

Unfortunately, Elizabeth developed brain metastasis. This made her question if what she did helped or not. She went on,

I have brain metastases since I've gone vegan, so I don't know if it's working. I don't know if it's helping. I don't know if it would be worse if I ate dairy. I don't know. I felt like it was worth a shot. It's healthy eating. So it's just my choice, but I don't know if it's helping.

In areas like this where there is no certainty about benefits or lack thereof for specific choices, the person can be left to grapple with the moral burden of the outcome of what they did or did not do. People with cancer are having to learn about their body and its physiology to make decisions, often with little data. Worse still, they feel the burden of the consequences of their decisions.

Another burden comes when the person starts to struggle to maintain strict expectations. For some, the notion of doing everything they can reaches a degree of moral obligation and almost becomes a burden. At that point, it can start to cause them to have guilt. Kim shared,

> I am trying to make sure that I'm staying healthy. I mean, my nutrition can probably improve a little bit more, I think, as far as diet, because then I feel like I have to be eating 100 percent healthy all the time. So, when I don't, there's a certain guilt element involved in it. Other than that, it's just trying to not obsess over it, because I'm an anxious person by nature even before I got cancer.

She realizes that her nutrition can be changed to make it better. She feels guilty if she does not eat well, and she tells herself that she has to eat healthily. This is when the matter becomes concerning. Rather than helping the person engage with the agency, it becomes a burden and an additional struggle.

Some participants, however, reflected critically on this concern for control and wanting to do anything, although the evidence to support effectiveness may be lacking.

Melissa took the privilege of explaining why her peers, the cancer patients, appear too focused on this or that matter. For her, it seems to be about having a sense of control, and that is why some choose a specific diet or supplement despite little or no evidence to back the choice. She remarked that people may be holding onto things that are not grounded in good reason, and when I asked for clarification, she added,

It's because they want to control, and they want to do something to make themselves better. They don't want to leave a stone unturned, that they didn't try every little thing that they could try. They also want to believe that there is something they can do. Then, there is also, I think, way more in the last fifteen or twenty years than there was before, a sort of hostility toward the medical profession.

I share the concerns Melissa expressed. Her thoughts and concerns are valid and well-grounded.

But how concerning is the desire to do everything, when many things do not change the course of the problem at hand?

And how bad is the hostility toward the medical profession? How can we address it?

I am left with troubling questions.

Exercising

J ust like the area of diet, people had a variety of choices around exercising. Exercising is generally considered part of what people choose to engage in when they think of health overall. Because the topic of health is salient among cancer patients, so is the topic of exercising. In the following pages, I will share reflections by patients on their choices around this area.

When dealing with cancer, some people chose to carry on with exercising the way they used to before they became ill. Some even started to do more as they try to provide better conditions for their bodies to deal with the illness.

Other people lost the capacity to exercise as they used to before their illness and that is what limited their exercising habits. Some did not think this area of health is as relevant to them because they considered maintaining reasonable weight as good enough or because they just want to not bother.

I Exercise

The participants did all kinds of exercise, and they did it for many reasons. I will share here about the forms of exercising and why people have chosen them.

Forms of exercise

The participants exercise in different ways. Some were running and going to the gym. Others chose activities that are less demanding on the body. Some had to reduce the frequency of their exercise so they could recover. Some went to exercise programs tailored to cancer survivors.

Some participants were fortunate to be able to make and maintain efforts at some form of exercising. For example, exercising was important for John. He explains,

> I tried to stay active. I tried to work out. Running has been a

little less, but before, I would do strength training; I would do weights.

Another person who had the privilege of continuing with physical activities was Amanda. She has always been active and continued to go to the gym.

> I keep going to the gym or playing golf pretty much every day. If I don't go to the gym or play golf, I walk in my neighborhood. So for me, getting up and being physically active is pretty important. I've taken up pickleball, added that to my little area of fitness, but I only play that in the winter. It just makes me feel good.

Exercising makes many people with cancer feel better, so being active has become essential. Some others have done exercises and gone to training that is tailored to survivors. Kim described her exercise routine:

> I've added other types of workouts to my daily exercise . . . I've been going to a facility that caters to cancer survivors as far as my workout. So, even my other classes, like strength training and things like that, are with other cancer survivors.

Some identified community programs for cancer survivors. Sharon was one of these:

> The exercise at the YMCA has been huge. I didn't know what the Leap Strong program was until I was diagnosed with cancer, and I recommend that to a lot of people. So that's probably the best example I could provide is the exercise and support through that program.

Some used to exercise more but never got back to it after the diagnosis, although they found alternative things to do to stay active. Nicole described this experience:

> I should have mentioned, before I had cancer, I was an avid bicyclist, and then I ended up giving that up with my

diagnosis. And then I have not gotten back up on the bicycle, and I'm not sure why that is, even though I'm feeling a lot better, I don't know. I think there's a fear of crashing maybe, and I'm not sure what that's about, but I haven't started riding my bicycle again.

Instead, Nicole identified other forms of activities. She explained,

I take dance classes. I can't dance full-on the way I used to because I get out of breath more quickly. I also sweat a lot more than I used to, and I think that's a function of the medicine. So, I take some dance classes, or as the weather gets worse, I think we'll go to the gym and I'll walk on the track or the treadmill and maybe do a stationary bike and do some weights. But right now, the weather is really nice, and so my husband and I will walk together for between two and five miles, depending on our schedule and depending on the weather and time of day we go out, but we walk a few times a week.

Many of these people never went back to exercising as before. Still, they carried on with alternative forms of exercise they thought were fit for them.

Why exercising

People were aware that exercising is vital for health. Some had exercised all their lives and continued to do so as their doctors recommended. Some of the participants think it is helping them fight the disease and is probably contributing to them faring well with disease control.

Some participants are aware that exercise is essential to health, and they never stopped, although they may do less. They attribute some of their fortunes in doing well to the fact that they continued to exercise. Larry is one of these people, and he said,

Exercise is important to health; always has been. I think that's one of the reasons I'm doing as well as I am is that I have not at all stopped exercising, although I do it much less.

People do what they are used to doing, especially when it is in line with what the oncologist recommends. John explained his exercising habits:

> Exercising was one thing my oncologist recommended, and that's actually what I was doing before that, so I just continued doing them.

Another person who has exercised all her life is Amanda:

> Exercising makes me feel good. I've exercised my whole life and been active my whole life. I get itchy if it's raining out and I can't get to the gym or go for a walk.

Exercising makes you feel good, and the participants exercised before their diagnosis. It is part of who the person is, and as Amanda said, they get itchy if they cannot exercise.

Many patients feel better when they do certain things routinely. This certainly applies to exercise. As Carol puts it, "Exercising makes me feel better. It is another way to keep cancer away. It also makes me feel better and look better."

Some feel they are getting stronger by exercising. Rebecca reflected this, saying, "Exercising helps me stay stronger. That's my big thing; it's just staying stronger with the back pain."

It helps them get stronger, and that is good.

I Exercise a Little or Not at All

Because of the illness, complications, or side effects of the medicine, some felt they had only a small capacity, or no capacity, to exercise. People have different reasons for not being able to engage in exercise even though they may want to.

This inability to exercise is a daily reminder of cancer for some. Jessica described it this way:

> That's probably the main daily reminder that I have cancer is I can't run again. I'm trying to walk every night in the neighborhood, and I have some hills, and they're very, very hard. Every day, that is a reminder that I have this terrible thing, you know, that I could probably run up this hill three years ago, and now I can't.

These patients may not be able to run although they wish they could, and that is what reminds them they have this disease. There were participants who had just finished rehab aimed at restoring some essential functional ability. Ashley is one of them:

> Exercising is not as routine as I would like it to be yet, and I consider just being able to do household tasks part of my healing because I couldn't do anything for a while. So I'm trying to break it down into small tasks and do the things that I can. I was discharged from physical therapy about five or six weeks ago, and I am on oxygen full time.

These people would still like to do more. However, their ability is so limited at this time that even doing household chores is an ambitious goal.

Another person who has no stamina to do much and is now doing more accessible forms of physical therapy as rehab is Stephanie. She explained,

> To be physically active as well, I do aquatic therapy. I still fatigue pretty easily. By doing the aquatic therapy, I'm not stiff as much. In the water, it's easier to move than it is on land, so I'm trying to build up so I can get back on to do on land—to do some of that. I used to run; I love to run, but I know right now is not the time. I won't have the stamina to do it.

Some people may barely have the capacity to do much and just manage to do physical therapy in aquatic settings. While they still want to be active, they find they have no stamina for more.

There are also others with even more severe limitations. Some had metastasis to the bones and then developed fractures that limited their capacity. Rebecca described this experience:

> I had the compression fracture in my back, so I started doing water exercise therapy to help make my back stronger, and that made me start being more conscious about exercising, and that kind of kickstarted my exercise and then movement and making me feel better with movement. I joined the YMCA program to get stronger. That seems to help with my spirit and my strength.

Another person who could not exercise because of problems in the spine is Christine. She explained,

> In terms of exercising, I can't really. I will never look at big exercises, but I exercise a little bit. I can't exercise because of my spine. So, the only thing they said I could do is to walk or run in a store mart. I walk when the weather is OK and when I can get myself out of the house.

People are doing what they can. However, fatigue can be extremely limiting. Donna has been dealing with this:

> I don't do much exercising except for walking around a little bit, but that is something that I want to add more to my life. It's just that I feel tired a lot of the time. That's an excuse because I've just never been much of an exerciser aside from like walking a little bit. Some time a few years ago, I was going to the gym and doing some swimming, but I've never been like a big health nut.

She feels tired, and some participants feel that their muscles are weak. For them, with the day-to-day running around, no room is left for more structured exercise. This is what Linda described:

> My exercise is just sort of living day-to-day, running around like crazy. Honestly, it's gotten a lot harder for me recently. I just, I haven't been feeling as well on the medicine. It's been a lot harder. I was running regularly up until about six months ago, but I couldn't do it anymore. My muscles are weak.

My lungs aren't quite as good. It's been harder for me, but some form of exercise, even if it's just walking, is always an improvement to me.

For many, day-to-day life consists of running around, which makes it difficult for them to retain the stamina to exercise much. As a result, some agreed that with their severe limitations, just getting up and moving is good enough. Mary voiced this viewpoint:

In regard to exercise, I don't do that daily, but I have found that just getting up and moving throughout the day, that tends to help with the muscle pain and the weakness and the achy joints, symptoms of that nature.

She does not do a regular exercise routine because she has muscle pain, which can afflict patients on specific treatments for this cancer. This incapacity can get so frustrating that they do little or nothing. Melissa described her experience in this regard:

Exercising? No. I don't do it; I don't believe in it. I mean, I do believe that exercise is good for you, but it was so frustrating always to have to be resting because it was impossible. Now, I can do things, so I get some exercise just by being able to do more activities with daily living, cleaning the house, anything.

To them, daily activities count as exercising. While they believe exercising is good, it is difficult to do when even maintaining daily activities is a challenge.

Of course, there were some people who were never big on exercising. Scott is one of them.

I did not exercise before. The old exercise I got before was doing yard work and work around the house, all the physical work. I don't particularly go out to exercise, other than taking the occasional walk with my wife when we had a dog. I try to stretch my legs and take a stroll from time to time. That's the main thing.

Some participants do little merely because they want to sit and not be bothered. Debora described this viewpoint:

> I walk the dogs. It's good exercise for them and me. I should be doing more because it's probably good for my body, keeping it healthier. Getting older and some things get me to thinking that I lose it or use it kind of thing. But sometimes, I just kind of feel that I can't be bothered or whatever; I don't—I'd rather sit and falter.

They realize that exercising keeps the body healthier and that they should do more. But conversely, they also assert that it is OK to sit and not exercise.

Donna delved into her sentiments in this regard:

> I want to live my life. I wasn't exercising a ton before. Yeah, I should have, but I wasn't dramatically overweight, and all my blood work was normal. My glucose, cholesterol, and blood pressure are all checked, and all are fine. I know that I need to lose a little bit of weight, but other than that, everything is healthy. So I feel like what I was doing was fine. I kind of still feel the same way if I am—whether it's cancer or not . . . like, being a model doesn't help fight my cancer. I feel like everything is fine. The doctor says, "Aside from cancer, you're healthy." So, what's the point of changing things dramatically?

Still, some continue trying to do more, and Jessica is among them:

> So my next step is I've got to get a handle on my diet and lose some weight. I think some of this stuff has caused me to gain weight, and it bothers me. If you were to ask me now, I wake up every day saying, OK, if I'm going to have to live with this cancer, then I need to get a hold of my diet, and I need to do something about the weight and exercise. I've got to be able to do more than a walk in my neighborhood. That's my next goal: What more can I do? I don't know, though, because I get out of breath just going up the stairs. So I don't know. I've

never been a yoga person, never done Pilates, but I've got to find something physical to replace that part that I gave up.

Ashley is another of the participants who has goals meant to transcend her limitations:

> I was discharged from physical therapy about five or six weeks ago because I met all the goals. Then I decided I wanted to do some more, so they are back with new goals. So I'm trying to just build the goals I have with daily exercises, and the physical therapist aid comes three times a week. I am on oxygen full time. I hope to get off of the oxygen because it limits what I can go out and do, and I would like to teach qigong again, and I would like to teach it without being hooked up to oxygen.

Many participants would like to do more than they currently can. However, like Ashley, mobility is so limited for many that even doing household chores has become an ambitious goal.

Complementary and Alternative Medicine

I n addition to making diet changes and exercising, people thought about or pursued a variety of Complementary and Alternative Medicine (CAM) practices. Through my interviews, I found that this part of health practices forms an essential component of what people do when they deal with an illness or just to maintain general good health.

Many people used these strategies before their illness, while others became open to these approaches after they became ill. Patients are correct. Medical doctors know very little about these approaches, and this research work was eye-opening for me as a physician.

What Kinds of CAM Do People Use?

I have divided the topics in this section according to categories of CAM therapy, including alternative medical systems (e.g., acupuncture), energy therapies (e.g., Reiki, qigong), exercise therapy (e.g., yoga), mind–body interventions (e.g., meditation, relaxation, mindfulness), nutritional therapies (e.g., supplements, vitamins, marijuana), and pharmacologic or biologic treatments (e.g., herbs, THC/CBD). Some participants have always used CAMs, while others became open to it after they developed cancer.

Alternative medical systems

Participants leveraged alternative medical systems to help manage many of their symptoms. In particular, acupuncture was popular among them. Amy explained, "I am going for acupuncture because I believe in that process, and so I found someone who was trained in China."

Nicole is also using acupuncture and said, "I started going to acupuncture mostly to treat anxiety. So, that's what I was doing at first, and it did help, it helped." Then Nicole was started on a new medicine that had side effects that troubled her. She explained,

When I started the medicine, I developed a pretty serious brain fog that wouldn't lift. I went around all summer feeling like I had molasses in the gears of my brain. Everything was slow, sort of like in sci-fi movies, when the spaceship slows down, and you hear that kind of woom–woom–woom–woom; that's how my brain felt. Then, I felt this terrible neuropathy, and it was painful at that time. Now it's not so painful, but then it was super painful. So they started treating me for those things at the acupuncture clinic, too, and those symptoms improved somewhat as well.

She described her first experience having acupuncture:

The first time I had an acupuncture treatment, I felt like I had kind of an out-of-body experience. It's like I was lifted out of the anxiousness and any aches and pains that I was having, any anxiety unraveled. When I go for the treatments now, the neuropathy eases and stays away that day and after acupuncture treatment for at least a week.

Nicole feels her struggles get worse when she does not get acupuncture as regularly as she would like. She explained,

Because I was traveling the past week, I didn't get in for my regular appointment, and I'll go this afternoon, but I can tell that I haven't been in over a week because the neuropathy is worse. I feel better after an acupuncture treatment; I feel more at ease in my body. I feel less anxious, and I was surprised. I went in skeptical, but I had seen the results my husband had gotten managing his back pain, and so I thought well, I'll try it.

For her, it helped ease anxiety.

Energy therapies

Some participants sought energy therapy. This became an essential part of the person's experience with cancer. It was part of a holistic approach that made sense of the illness and provided a framework for understanding. Among these practices, the most common were Reiki and qigong.

One person in particular, Robert, found a Reiki practitioner to help with his experience. He explained,

> Immediately, I did a lot of spiritual work, and I wanted to come clean to myself about all of the things in the past and to start loving myself. So I went to a Reiki practitioner to help me figure that out. I wanted them to help me to have a true love for myself so that I could start healing properly.

For those who seek Reiki, it is often part of the spiritual work. They get coaching from the practitioner.

Another person who found Reiki to be useful is Christine.

> There's like a club for Reiki in New York near my house. It's for people with cancer. I can't tell you much about it. I don't understand it. It has something to do with energy. I don't know how it works, but it feels good.

In addition to Reiki, another energy treatment is qigong. Ashley noted, "I do my qigong practice. I'm starting to put that back in."

Ashley has taught qigong and focused on energy work for years. For her, it is part of healthy living. But now she is on oxygen full time. Her hope is to get off the oxygen so she can teach qigong again and continue to pursue a higher degree for teaching it.

Exercise therapy

Exercise therapy, especially yoga, seems to be particularly popular. Interestingly enough, different people got different things from yoga. Some found in it a place to move their body and stretch, others focused on the meditation aspect, while some found transformation in the experience.

Some people enjoyed the aspects that relate to stretching and exercising the body. Elizabeth said, "I've done some yoga stretching classes with friends." Others do yoga because it is enjoyable and helps with strengthening.

Stephanie elaborated on this point:

> I'm going to get involved in a yoga class. Well, it'll help with strengthening, stress release, and it's something that I always enjoyed. I do it to be physically active as well.

For some, yoga had always been part of their life as a form of physical activity and as a healthy routine. Samantha explained,

> Yoga is a big thing in my life. I've been doing yoga for twenty-five years, and it's been hard for me to not be able to do it because I had a daily yoga practice for years. There was a time when I was too weak to do it. So the fact that I'm able to do it again to some extent gives me satisfaction. I know I'll never be able to do it as I used to, but it feels good to see that I can progress instead of regress in something physical like that.

Others started doing yoga after they developed cancer and tried to find an exercise strategy. Yoga changed their conception of being active and working out. Richard touched on this point:

> I had to change my perspective of what working out was. Yoga never fit that definition before lung cancer. I wouldn't have had the patience to even think of it as exercise. The way I see it now, I don't need to sweat to give my body the benefit of exercise, literally. I don't need to be panting so hard, I'm killing myself. Like, I grew up playing football, running track, and doing all that. So the philosophy behind yoga for me was that if I'm stretching areas of my body, if I'm getting blood flow to muscles that typically don't get exercised during running or lifting weights, then I'm pushing my body to its optimum.

Yoga, for him, gives the benefits of exercising and has had a positive impact on his mind-set. It felt to him as if he didn't need to do strenuous exercises if he could do yoga instead, and that changed how he thinks about exercising.

Some participants have done yoga in the past but now cannot do it as intensely, like Nicole:

> Yoga is something I've been practicing for twenty years. It's
> something that we do as a family as well, and yoga has a
> profound effect on the nervous system. I've always used it to
> help myself be calm, to cope with anxiety. I also have some
> issues with my back, which I've had since I was a teenager,
> and so yoga helps me manage those problems and strengthen
> my spine. We also use yoga as a tool for meditation, and that
> also helps. I use it to manage chronic back issues but also to
> address anxieties.

Nicole practiced yoga with her daughter, who is a yoga instructor. With
her illness and its progression now, Nicole has only been able to do a little of
what she calls "restorative yoga." She enjoys it and finds it helpful for easing
her anxieties.

Mind–body interventions

Many participants also practiced meditation and mindfulness,
approaching mind–body connections from different viewpoints and for
different reasons.

Some participants chose to approach their illness holistically, and that
meant caring for both the body and the mind. John explained,

> I started to take care of myself in the whole aspects, including
> mentally and spiritually. I try to meditate as much as I can
> daily, so I have a practice, a meditation practice. I sit there,
> and I try to observe my body and sensations. So one technique
> I use is to focus on each of my senses separately—what I hear,
> what I smell, what my skin feels—and I try to focus on that
> instead of focusing on my thoughts. Another technique that
> I use is to just observe my thoughts without reacting to them
> or with a new reaction. I observe what goes through my mind
> knowing that they're just thoughts, that they don't mean
> anything unless I react. That is how I do it.

For John, meditation has helped to give him peace.

Some of the people had practiced meditation before becoming ill, which is the case for Cynthia: "I do meditation, but I did that before I got sick. I find that it's even more valuable to me now."

However, others only began meditating after their diagnosis. Brandon describes his experience:

> One thing I tried to do every day and started right about when I was diagnosed is meditation. I do guided meditation, maybe for twenty minutes at a time. It's beneficial for keeping me grounded in the present and not getting overwhelmed or becoming anxious about things that are in the past or the things that might happen in the future. I still have the usual anxieties and worries, but I feel like I'm better able to cope with things like that.

Meditation, especially guided meditation, can help some people, like Brandon, feel less worry. Other participants pointed out the benefits of meditation for dealing with emotions. John describes this aspect:

> I think meditation has helped me a lot to deal with the emotional aspect of it. I'm just more accepting of everything, and it helps me be in the present, more in the moment and not so much caught up in the past or what could happen in the future. It released a lot of the anxiety, I believe, a lot of the depression that could come with it. You know, I do experience some anxiety and depression, but it doesn't overpower me.

A common benefit of meditation is the way it helps people to focus on living more in the moment. Meditation can even help some people come to terms with death or in dealing with the potential for the disease to progress, as it did for Justin:

> I meditate, which is a way that I find the entire calmness and dealing with the stress of this entire thing. I've gotten over the days when I used to have scan anxiety, with a lot of concerns.

I was not sure what I would find when I would go back for the results of the scan. That used to keep me up at night for quite a bit, days on end, until the appointment, and I would not be able to focus with the family. So the meditative side has helped to handle that.

Justin also shared how meditation has helped him transform his perspective, the way he looks at things.

After a diagnosis like this, where mortality hits you in the face, it naturally raises the question of what is beyond me. And I'm an analyst, so I research and I research to a point where I realized meditation is the key. I wake up, and the first thing that I realize is I'm breathing. I don't need anything after that. I'm completely satisfied, and that has made a huge impact on just how I feel, how I walk, how I think, and people around me in my professional work know that, even if they haven't met me before. They talk to me for years on the phone, and they say, "Wow, there's something about you." I tell them these are the only things I've done that are different, that they've made a complete change to my entire existence, giving me an understanding on the mortality side that I've now come to terms with death. I now come to terms with this diagnosis. And I understand that tomorrow morning, I may go for a scan and everything could unravel, and it's a horrible situation. But it's easier said than done, but I have—I want a power behind me now, strength behind me for my meditation that this is the journey of life.

Meditation has given Justin calmness and acceptance. While many people recognize that meditation can be helpful, they do not practice it often. Debora noted this tendency:

I should meditate, but I don't. Meditation helps to calm. Keep it down. I should do more of that because it's very calming and it's good for the spirit. But it's hard for me to sit. My mind races; I start thinking about bringing my mind back to it, and it doesn't come easily to me.

Related to meditation, and often practiced in conjunction with it, is mindfulness. Some people had specific mindfulness practices. Being mindful in every moment is something they try; it is a practice in everyday activities and a mind-set. Linda explained,

> I do try to do a mindfulness practice, even if that means being present in my day-to-day activities. Even if I don't take time out to meditate, I'll try to do things mindfully. For example, in the morning, brushing my teeth, instead of planning my day and figuring out what I'm going to wear or whatever it is, I try to only brush my teeth. It's a mindful practice. Sometimes, at things like that, sometimes it just includes the kids. We try to have gratitude practice with dinner. We'll go to the table and talk about the things that we're feeling grateful for that day. Things like that.

The practice of gratitude is trendy and is also related to mindfulness and being present in the moment. Melissa also found mindfulness therapy to be helpful, and she appreciates that.

> That was the smartest thing that I did. That gave me the most support. And they had lots of systems there, too. They had mindfulness-based stress reduction, and it's wonderful. They teach you mindfulness. They have little classes, but then they had this one that went on for nine weeks, and it was three hours a week, and then a whole day at the end. You really learned to meditate and how to use your breathing when you get stressed and how just to develop a mindfulness practice, which I never really did before. But I use the techniques of breathing and stress and all that other jazz. They were wonderful. That was a real resource. I had a private therapist I went to in the beginning, too. Now I go if there's a crisis, when I had the recurrence or stuff like that. But I don't go regularly. They helped me greatly with tailoring the care because the worst problem that I had was fatigue, and I was just very frustrated

that I couldn't do all the things I want to do and was spending so much time lying down. And for that, they were very helpful.

Nutritional therapies

Some of the participants took supplements or vitamins, as well as other nutritional therapies. When they see a patient with cancer, the public are often generous in their recommendations regarding supplements. Some patients were open to taking them, while others were skeptical.

Some participants tried many supplements, like Sarah:

> Well, I've tried lots of things. I do take a lot of supplements. I wasn't allowed to in the beginning because they didn't want anything to interfere with the cancer treatment. But yes basically, I take essential oils every day, vitamins, and mineral supplements.

Some of them have come to realize that they take a lot of supplements. Like diet, this is an area where others are often generous with making suggestions. Mary described that,

> When I was first diagnosed, I got all these suggestions, "Oh, you need to be taking these supplements." I was taking supplements, and it had just gotten me to a point where I was just taking it because somebody's telling me to take it other than my doctor.

Mary finally, at one point, realized that she should not take supplements just because others suggested them. The doctor in me wonders why people like to play the doctor's role and whether they are entitled to make such recommendations.

Some participants are taking vitamins, like Elizabeth:

> I'm vegan for five months. I did not realize I needed B12, and you don't get it from anything but meat. You have to supplement it. My oncologist said I could take a B12 supplement.

Elizabeth's oncologist had made the recommendation against her being vegan, but she had dismissed the oncologist's opinion. When her hair started to fall out, she resorted to B12 supplements.

Another participant who was taking vitamins and supplements is Carol:

> I was taking supplements even before. I take multivitamins; I take calcium. I take other things. I am continuing to take them, but unfortunately, I had to add more and more supplements to my daily routine because of the side effects of the medicine. Now, I am taking L-lysine because sometimes I get mouth sores and they become painful. I had mouth sores before, but, I understand that this is one of the side effects. So I am taking L-lysine now. I am taking biotin and silica because I want my hair to grow back. I was not taking that before.

Like Carol, some patients take supplements to counter the side effects of the treatment if the supplement is something people have recommended and that the oncologist does not disagree with. Patients will often try whatever they hear about to put themselves in the best position.

Pharmacologic and biologic treatments

A few participants consider herbal management to be part of their treatment. This strategy has helped some with symptoms related to their illness and helped others deal with some of their struggles. CBD was a topic of interest for me, and I explore it at some depth in the following pages.

In terms of herbal management in general, some people considered it to be part of their care plan. Justin explained,

> Something I've found helpful to manage my condition is herbal management. Physicians are not trained to provide you with a holistic approach to medicine other than medicine itself, and so I take herbal supplements.

Notably, in many cases, participants recognized that they should check with their oncologist before adding supplements of any sort.

Some participants use CBD as part of their health-related activities to deal with cancer. And among that group, some of them came to using CBD based on elaborate theories, such as happened with Sarah:

> A friend of mine's mom had eye cancer, and she reached out to me. And she was like, "Hey, have you considered taking CBD oil?" And I was like, "Ugh, I don't know if I want to do that or not." And as I started researching it, I was like, "Why wouldn't I take this? Our body is designed for this; we have a system and receptors," so I started taking CBD oil.

Although Sarah recognizes that she primarily uses CBD oil because life sucks and she wants a good night of sleep, she explained the elaborate theory of the cannabinoid system:

> We have a system in our body; it's set up and called the cannabinoid system. We have these receptors throughout our body that accept this oil. The idea is that the CBD with THC, when you take them together, one keeps the cancer cells from proliferating, and the other one causes cell mitosis. So again, with my cancer specifically, I'm not sure if there is a connection there.

Sarah and I were having this conversation over Zoom. I wonder if she felt uncomfortable explaining these things to me, a physician, and she stopped herself. She laughed, and I reassured her with a smile. She went on,

> I'm going to take it anyway. When life sucks, it's OK to take some CBD oil. It helps relax me, and I sleep at night.

I could not agree more. When life sucks, it is OK to use CBD, if that is what you choose and prefer.

For other participants, CBD helps with symptoms. Nancy said,

> I'll take CBD oil, which is made from hemp. It helps with pain and anxiety. The CBD oil, it's made from hemp, so it doesn't have any THC in it. It doesn't have any psychoactive drugs that give you that high feeling. I like it. It helps me with

my pain. I take the CBD oil under my tongue, the tincture. It works OK. Not as great as Advil. But I have such a sensitive stomach for my medication, I can't take Advil anymore. So, yeah, the CBD oil, it's great. They say it's also helped with anxiety. I haven't noticed if it helped me with my anxiety. [Laughs]

Others also use CBD for pain, although the results are varied. Carol was one who tried this:

When I was having symptoms from the recurrence, I thought I had sciatica. I had tried to do some edibles. I tried to ease the pain, but it didn't work. It worked for a while.

Others use marijuana simply because they use it. Lisa stated it succinctly: "I am a marijuana user." And that is that.

Participants who tried CBD and did not continue were often bothered by some effects of THC/CBD, such as nausea or feeling high. Debora had that experience:

I tried to do CBD/THC. Even though I used very little, like a little rice kernel of it. You're supposed to try to titrate up to like one gram a day, which is like an enormous amount, that's where they say it's therapeutic for cancer. I don't know. Just that little tiny thing, I took it at night, it just made me feel nauseous and high, and I don't know, dizzy. I didn't like the feeling. I never took drugs when I was younger, so I'm not into that. I didn't like the feeling, and so I stopped taking it.

These kinds of side effects of CBD/THC can be a limiting factor when people do not like how it feels.

There continues to be a stigma around using CBD. This is what Rebecca alluded to:

The CBD oil, I've been very reluctant on that. I think part of that is my history as a law enforcement officer. Yes, I've seen people use it, and I've seen results with them. I just have felt like my symptoms have not been that extreme that I would need it at this point. But I try to say never say never, because you never know when you'll be in the situation where maybe that might help. But then I haven't gone down that road yet on CBD oil.

Some participants were just very skeptical about the use of these treatments. Andrew noted some of the ideas that are spread among patient groups:

> I go to this chat room, and people are there to exchange information about treatments and side effects, and I often find that I have the best information that's scientifically based. There's a ton of stuff that goes back and forth with people who say, "Try CBD oil; insert it anally," or something like that, I mean, I was like, "Are you kidding me? What are you smoking? What makes you think that is going to do you any good?" Or turmeric, that's the other one. "I've been taking turmeric, and I survived this long. Therefore, it's turmeric that's keeping me alive." And then I go, "It might have something to do with that cancer treatment you're taking, too. I wonder if that had anything to do with it!"

I verified that there exists CBD oil that is inserted anally, in a suppository form. For Andrew, this is about misguided information, and he is suspicious of the reasoning some people provide when attributing improvement to these supplements even though they are also already on active treatment. He finds the idea of using CBD in its different forms ridiculous, and he laughs at our human absurdity. He goes so far as considering CBD a ridiculous idea and an insult to intelligence.

Remarks on the Choices around Health Actions

Many of the strategies already mentioned around diet and complementary approaches are, for some patients, not considered "complementary" or "alternative" at all but are, rather, the main mode of self-care. For some people, it is Western medicine that is "alternative." The choice for this or that strategy is often shaped not only by the person's philosophy in life but, interestingly enough, also by the person's access to health care. Many people have limited access to health care because they have no insurance. As a result, they focus on staying healthy as opposed to receiving health care when they become ill. These health care choices are not without consequences.

Some participants made non-western medicine their main mode of health care. Ashley is an example. She was a student of Chinese medicine and a certified qigong instructor and practitioner. Ashley had studied nutrition and herbs for many years and "didn't use allopathic medicine much at all. I did a lot of self-care." Her career for over twenty years was "working within the healing world, doing massage therapy, reflexology, and different kinds of energy work." Ashley felt she had been reasonably healthy until the cancer diagnosis. She explained,

> In fact, I think that's why I was in such an advanced state, because it just couldn't make sense to me that I could be sick with something as big as cancer.

When Ashley was diagnosed with cancer, she became more open to allopathic medicine. She explained,

> I've always said that there's a place for Western medicine, and I will always honor and respect it and use it if I need to. Well, now I need it, so that's what I'm doing. When you're faced with a sudden terminal diagnosis, you're more open to what might work for you. I know that there's been a lot of advances in cancer treatment over the last few years. So I just decided to be open to whatever suggestions they had and evaluate it to see what the best approach for me was.

Ashley took pride in being a "very independent person." She focused on health and not on disease, on her body's ability to heal itself rather than on taking medications. But there is another side to Ashley's story, and learning about this aspect opened my eyes to how people make health choices. Ashley had limited access to health care in the past because she did not have health insurance. She explained,

> Not having health insurance is pretty intimidating, and you just want to try to do everything that you can to keep yourself healthy without having to have an intervention.

Like millions of Americans today, Ashley did not have health insurance most of her adult life. Not having insurance shaped her health choices. She said,

> When you don't have that, and you want to be healthy, and you want to be independent and be in charge . . . I wanted to be responsible for my own well-being and my own health.

Without insurance, you feel that you must stay healthy because it is expensive to get sick. Ashley went on,

> The thought of having to go to the emergency room or to the hospital and get a CT scan is scary. I mean, your first thought is, "How am I going to pay for that?" and it's pretty intimidating. Just struggling with the financial part of it is huge.

Because Ashley was self-employed, she could not afford health coverage, even when she turned sixty-five and became eligible for Medicare. She noted,

> Once I turned sixty-five, I found out that Medicare isn't free. There's a premium, and it comes out of your social security check, and at that point, we were pretty much retired with only a little social security income. We couldn't afford to take another $200 a month out of that. Nobody ever told us that the state's health welfare could pay the premium because of our low income.

Ashley's attitude toward health was shaped by her philosophy and access to health care, but still, she wishes she had been more open to seeking medical care earlier. She reflected on her position during our conversation.

> The only thing that I wish I had done differently is that I would have understood the symptoms and had more curiosity and pursued a diagnosis at an earlier date.

What happened to Ashley also happens to many people because the symptoms of lung cancer are not easy to recognize, and the possibility of getting ill with such a devastating disease does not come to the mind. The person, however, is always left to wonder if being more curious and seeking medical help at an earlier date would have made a difference.

Not different from Ashley's experience and questions were those of John. John's narrative centers on how healthy eating keeps the person healthy; he believes in the power of healthy food. For him, it was not about a specific diet but rather about a *balanced* healthy diet that helped. He always does meal prep on the weekends, which makes it easier for him to eat healthily throughout the week. Before he became ill, he started a business that focuses on assisting people in staying healthy by supplying them with prepared meals of good nutritious value for the week. It was because he enjoyed it himself that he wanted to share it through his business. He explained,

> I decided to try to help other people with this technique, and so I began a business that tries to teach others how to be more efficient in the kitchen and how to meal prep for themselves.

John started promoting his ideas, and he got people's attention. Then something happened. He explained,

> I started having symptoms four months before diagnosis. I noticed some tightness in my chest, and I thought it was a hernia. I self-diagnosed at that time because I was unemployed. I was self-employed, so I didn't have health insurance. I just googled the symptoms, and I concluded that it was a hernia. So I just disregarded it, and it did get a little better.

Then his disease progressed and presented itself through a loss of voice while he was promoting his ideas about a healthy diet. He added,

> A few months after my early symptoms, I had a presentation
> related to my business. It was a marketing event, and at the
> beginning of the event, I asked how many people in the
> audience either know someone or are themselves affected by
> cancer. I was talking about nutrition and how nutrition can
> help us prevent disease, and ironically, that's the day that I lost
> my voice. After my presentation, I couldn't speak anymore.

John was in another state for the event. He also had terrible back and
chest pain. He tried to "self-medicate, just try to take care of it on my own
because I was out of state, and I was also not insured." But after he had
returned home, he could not take it anymore, and he was admitted to the
hospital via the emergency room.

John was diagnosed with stage IV lung cancer as he was hospitalized
and, the irony is that diet did not prevent his cancer.

The fact that diet did not prevent his cancer has troubled John, as he
revealed during our conversation. After the diagnosis, John has continued to
hold the belief that nutrition is essential. He continues to be "a firm believer
in the power of nutrition and how food can heal." He wishes he would have
received more support in that area from the start, right after his diagnosis.
He did not appreciate that he was initially told that he "could eat whatever;
that I should just try to maintain my weight." After his illness, he reshaped
his volunteer work around diet to help cancer survivors. He explained,

> I do send out meal plans with recipes and shopping lists that
> cancer patients can use to help them with their nutrition.
> That's meaningful to me because I feel like I'm helping people
> in my situation.

He also started seeing a nutritionist at his cancer center and a naturopath
because he appreciates a holistic approach.

I have a position on this matter as a physician. I mean what I say when I say that I have no problem with individuals privileging self-care or care from alternative frameworks. But I can see the limits of alternative approaches. When someone carries on attempting to self-heal beyond the space where self-healing works, it delays them seeking care that does work. Also, when someone tries alternative strategies that have no proven effects *instead* of what is effective, the desired outcomes are jeopardized.

For some patients, the illness changed their position on how to best care for oneself. Some became open to Western medicine. Similarly, those who believe diet prevents and cures cancer may have their claims challenged when they develop cancers themselves. While it is good to put the responsibility for self-care on the person and to advise people to live healthily, I worry that people may be burdened by the claims made by some regarding the effectiveness of some health choices in preventing death, curing cancer, and ending chronic diseases without these claims having sufficient evidence to back them up.

Living healthily is good. People can enjoy a diversity of health practices that have immediate and long-term positive effects. These practices, however, are not going to necessarily cure cancer nor prevent it in the way some people with passion talk about the matter. At least, we do not know that to be true at this point.

In the end, what kept these the participants here alive was not this or that diet or health choice; instead, it was receiving targeted chemotherapy. Before these treatments, people used to die from advanced lung cancer in only a few months. Now, those who are eligible for these treatments are living for years.

Taking Targeted Chemotherapy

The one health action all of these patients did was taking medicine for their cancer. They all were on targeted chemotherapy, and they did so for similar reasons: to reduce the cancer or to keep it stable. They know their disease is incurable, but they also know they can keep on living as long as the medicine is working. They also know that their treatment, what is keeping them alive, will eventually stop working. Nonetheless, they hope that science will bring newer treatments at a rapid pace and in time for them.

The medicine works. It reduces the cancer's size and keeps the disease under check. When I asked Donna about the reason for taking the medicine, she explained,

> I want to reduce the cancer that I have in my body and keep it under control, and my hopes are that the medication will shrink all of the tumors. My goal is to eliminate my cancer. Now, I know that's a lofty goal, but that's my goal because I want to live. I don't want to die from cancer. I'm too young to die, and I'm thirty-seven now. I'm not ready for that.

She holds on to the hope that the medicine will shrink all of her tumors. She recognizes that eliminating the cancer may be close to impossible, but she wants to be hopeful and at least get a reduction in the size of the cancer. She wants to live, and she only lives if the cancer shrinks.

The desire to stay alive and to fight the cancer was similar for Carol, who explained, "I am taking the medicine because I want to stay alive, and I want to kill the cancer." It was also a no-brainer for Rebecca, who explained, "I take it to help control and keep my cancer stable; that's how I explain it in my mind."

The patients have no doubts that their medicines are working, and they have many reasons to believe that is true. They were going on living at a point where many patients with lung cancer would have died quickly in the past. When I asked Melissa why she takes the medicine, she replied,

The targeted therapy? Oh, well, my uncle died in two months with lung cancer, and here I am, five and a half years later, talking to you and raising a child and having friends and going on vacations and living life.

The evidence is clear from a comparison. In the past, lung cancer patients died quickly, but today, the person can keep on living—*with* a good quality of life.

The medicine works, and there is no doubt about that.

Patients also do not doubt is that their medicines are destined to stop working at some point, that the cancer will eventually develop resistance to the drugs and then grow without control. This is what Debora referred to when she explained, "I take the medicine because it works. I mean, it's going to keep me alive until my cancer resists it." The medicine keeps working—until it stops working.

Developing resistance to treatment and having progression of disease are every cancer patient's nightmares. For these patients, it is particularly difficult given that they know science is making progress. It is just a matter of staying alive until a next lifeline comes to the scene. Katherine described this,

Well, with the targeted therapy, I know that eventually, the cancer will mutate and continue to grow, and at that point, there are a couple of things that I can do. But it's like, you know the old game, Frogger, where you are trying to cross the river, and you jump on the rock, and then you need the next rock to come up before the one that you're standing on sinks? That's what it's like. I'm standing on my rock, and I know it's going to sink, and I know there's half of one foot sinking while maybe another rock is starting to come up. I want that next rock so I can make it across.

Patients realize that the current treatment is going to fail, and then they have a few other options, which will all eventually fail. Regardless, they continue hoping that science will progress faster than their disease.

My Health Actions

It is only fair for the reader to ask what it is that I am doing in the area of health. I will share some about that here. But before doing that, I want to share some reflections on how I became ill.

As I mentioned before, I have dealt with inflammatory bowel disease for years. This condition gave me gastrointestinal troubles. I would have stomach pain and bad diarrhea. Due to the nature of this illness, I had episodes of bad flare-ups, but even at baseline, I struggled with bothersome symptoms.

One of those flare-ups landed me in the hospital. When I left, I was on steroids and started to struggle with the side effects from that. Not all of the side effects were bad. One, for example, was having a tremendous amount of energy. I wrote papers and signed up for the PhD that I completed in the years afterward. Other, less pleasant, side effects included not sleeping well at night, being hostile and irritable, and gaining a lot of weight.

I came off steroids and switched to medicine that suppressed my immune system. Less than two years after, I developed Stage 4 lung cancer.

We know that cancers develop as random mutations that switch on irregular cell production. The immune system usually keeps that irregularity under check. It was plausible that my immune system was not working effectively, at least in part, due to the treatment I had been on.

Every patient with cancer reflects on how they came to develop the disease. Many look at their past for what they have done or what has happened to them and try understand how they ended up with this nasty disease. When, we, lung cancer patients tell people about our cancers, they almost always ask us if we smoked. People want to explain this disease and, if possible, find a reason to think they are immune from it.

During my conversations with the participants in this work, almost half the people started their self-introduction by affirming that they had done nothing to cause this illness. Many would assert that they did their best before the disease to eat healthily and to exercise.

There is the fear that they may have brought cancer upon themselves. There is a stigma associated with smoking, and people who do or did smoke get blamed for their lung cancer.

This stigma really sucks.

I am sharing my reflection to say that this is not fair to those people who develop cancer, even the ones who have smoked. It is not fair to any of us.

I made a choice. I went on an immunosuppressant so I could keep going with my life and maintain a level of health that is conducive to doing good things. People make those choices. People struggle with physical and mental health and choose to deal and cope with these struggles using this or that strategy. I decided to take medicine. Some people want to smoke. Some do none of those. Yet cancer can and does happen to any of us, although some people may be more predisposed to it than others because of the choices that they have made.

My experience with being a cancer patient taught me to be a doctor who does not judge his patients for any health decision they make or even if they live in oblivion to the consequences of their passive choices. Still, I want, as a doctor, to support people so they can make the best decisions possible—and to forgive themselves when things go wrong.

The heart of the matter is that it is difficult to predict who will develop any specific cancer. It is not easy to avert them, either.

What I am saying should not be taken as a license for people to do whatever they want and to shirk the responsibility. It is true that if someone avoids smoking, they will reduce their chances of getting cancer. That is true, and that is how I would recommend people think about the matter. It is also true that if people eat one thing or another, it may boost their chances of developing related conditions. But this relationship between what we choose to do and our diseases should never be part of the conversation that would deter someone from accessing support and empathy.

Also, this relationship should never be the focus of the person who is burdened with the disease. It could consume the person from the inside out with guilt and self-blame. That is not fair. Instead, we could think about now. Now that we have this disease, what can we do to optimize the conditions?

I came to terms with the fact that cancer is what I have, and I am not going to reverse it, but I can do what I can to live as healthily as possible while I am alive because it is good and may help optimize my chances of staying well.

Now let me share what I do in the area of health.

As part of doing healthy things, and because I am a physician who advises people to watch their weight and diet, I do pay attention to staying in a reasonable range when it comes to my weight. I also try not to obsess about it out of vanity. I want to love myself and to forgive myself as well.

As a physician who is also mindful of recommending and doing what has evidence of efficacy and not spending time over what is not fact-based, I tend to focus on eating a variety of food in moderation rather than making any extreme diet choices. That is my preference as a person as well. A variety of foods are enjoyable, and I do not want to forbid myself having any particular thing, especially if there is no convincing evidence that abstaining from this or that would make me live longer or better. (There is the moral argument, of course, for becoming vegetarian, but that is not the topic here.)

If the future brings evidence to support some forms of extreme diets, I would also weigh the benefit against the cost of changing my lifestyle and will judge the mental energy I would spend on the matter.

My relationship with exercising has varied throughout my experience with illness. I was working out when I first noticed that I was not breathing well. From that standpoint, exercising was maybe my lifesaver. Had I been sedentary, I might not have discovered my limited capacity (because of cancer spreading around my lungs) for probably another few months. I could also reflect that I may have started working out again because I was not feeling well due to the cancer already developing. I was probably rebuilding my endurance because I was feeling ill as a result of cancer.

Either way, exercising is essential and beneficial.

Early on in my illness, I could not exercise much. My lungs lost their compliance, and for a while, I had liters of fluids around them. Almost a year later, I was by myself, walking in the street in the middle of the night, and I panicked. To get to a "safe place," I started running. I discovered that I was *able* to run, and I started working out again.

The medicine I am on gave me muscle pain and fatigue. I struggled to find the right balance. Exercising helped my energy level, but too much exercising would drain my energy and result in pain. In addition to working my day job, I was then working on my PhD dissertation and also interviewing people for this project. I had to choose whether to maintain the little energy I have so I could write or spend my energy exercising. It was a hard decision. I was also probably overwhelmed with my struggle, and that had drained a lot of my mental energy.

I feel fortunate now that I started back on an exercise regimen where I use the gym for bicycling, elliptical training, and weight training at least every other day. I started doing that about five weeks ago, and it has been excellent. I have made a conscious decision to build time into my schedule for self-care.

I say I feel fortunate because it is not all my doing. My disease has not yet taken my capacity to exercise. I am also in good mental health. It is an enormous help to me. I am in a good position in life. I have already written a paper about this project, and I am finishing this book. I can take it easy now.

I am able to slow down and take care of myself.

Other things I have tried include yoga, a couple of times. I enjoyed it, and it helped relax my mind. It even led to the common euphoric effects, experienced by the seasoned yogis, of feeling healthy and wanting to drink green juices immediately afterward. I had that happen to me twice.

I used meditation when I was struggling mentally and emotionally by listening to guided meditation tapes, and they helped relax my mind.

I take vitamin D because my level was low, and I had fatigue. I felt it might have helped with my fatigue, but it's hard to tell. I probably did many other things at the same time to help with fatigue, such as exercising, paying attention to sleeping more, and seeking others' emotional support.

Let me say a few words on my own primary treatment. I take targeted chemotherapy in a pill form. I started on a medicine called crizotinib six weeks after my cancer diagnosis. But when a study came out in June of 2017 showing that a newer agent, called alectinib, is better than my crizotinib in terms of expected survival and the prevention of brain metastasis, my oncologist suggested that I switch to it. I have been on this newer medicine since the fall of 2017. I foresee that I will end up changing to other agents or chemotherapy in the future, when my current treatment fails, but I am hopeful it can work for a long time. I also hope that research will find more treatment options while I am still alive.

As a final comment, I want to never judge any person for whatever they want to do in the area of health and well-being. I hope to provide some insight from different people's experiences, and I also want to call attention to positions that might be extreme in one direction or another. Ultimately, I want to shed light on the space where someone can enact their agency to do a little more if they want to and can, not necessarily to cure the illness but rather to live in the way they want to live.

So this book is not about what a person should do to live better with cancer. This is only about what some people with cancer are doing. If you want to know what you could or should do in terms of your health, speak to your doctor, or do your own research using trusted, evidence-based health resources.

Part Four:

**COPING WITH
THE STRUGGLE**

I asked the participants, "How are you coping with cancer?" and I clarified by adding, "How do you deal with stress?" I aimed to inquire what these people do to be able to carry on with cancer and what they do to manage the stress that works for them.

Cancer shifts many aspects of a person's life. It is an experience of struggle. The existential threat also comes with a challenge to everything that makes the person who they are. The person's roles in life shift and so do the relationships they form with people around them. Also, the person's understanding of their life's purpose changes with the uncertainty of their prognosis.

Living with cancer is uncharted territory for those experiencing the illness. This novelty is especially real for people with lung cancer with oncogenic alterations. There are positive prospects that came with targeted chemotherapies. There is hope. Still, there are many daunting uncertainties. Patients are living the experience of a struggle in trying to find meaning and maintain strength. They also have to answer many questions related to ordinary day-to-day matters.

Cancers abruptly disrupt a person's biography. They create a discontinuity. The uncertainty in the lives of these forty individuals and those living with similar conditions makes their experiences particularly challenging. They do not know how long they will live and cannot conceptualize priorities the way people who are not sick do.

People who expect to live a long life prioritize future goals around expanding their horizons and seeking life opportunities. Those perceiving an imminent boundary on their life resort to the warmth of emotions that come with established relationships. We learned that from psychological theories. The forty people in this book swing back and forth between the two attitudes.

There is the *hope* to carry on, and that new drugs will make it possible for the person to live a long time, and the person wants to do what ordinary people do. But there is also the *fear* that cancer will progress quickly, and there will be no time to even say goodbye to their loved ones. These are two attitudes that build on this hope or that fear. There is also the attitude that unites the two: living an intentional life while being mindful of time limits and while doing what is meaningful with those people the person cares most about.

We have seen that before, in the first two chapters, when we read about people finding meaning and building resilience. In the following pages, I will share reflections on what people are doing in the day-to-day to cope with their struggle and their stress. These are actions that people do to maintain a sense of purpose and of their identity.

Unsurprisingly, they did different things.

To cope, people maintained their agency by volunteering and doing advocacy work. They also held onto relationships that were meaningful to them, such as those with family and friends.

In addition, they have shifted their frameworks around to better align with what is conducive to carrying on. For example, they attempt to redirect their attention, try to be positive, or use humor.

Some have coped by learning about their cancer and how to manage it. Others have coped by living life in the here and now.

Finally, some people needed extra rest and found that to be what helped them cope.

Maintaining Agency

S ome of these people cope by preserving agency, which meant different things. For some, it was in advocacy work. For others, it was volunteering and helping other survivors by providing mentorship at times. Some wanted to participate in research to move things forward for their own and others' treatments.

Advocacy

Rather than dealing with cancer as an individual's personal struggle, some of the participants found social aspects to their experience. Having the disease and suffering connected them to the plight of other cancer patients.

They understand others' experience because, in that other person's struggle, they see aspects of their own. They also realize how things ought to be if we want to provide better conditions for those with cancer to survive their struggle. They are conscious of what is good and what is right, and they are sensitive, with disdain, to what is not right and not good.

Furthermore, with cancer, they reclaim their voice. As they reflect on who they are, they become aware of what they stand for. In other words, they become advocates.

For some, advocacy is an opportunity to be around people with a similar struggle. This was Stephanie, who explained, "I do a lot of advocacy work for lung cancer; it's more so networking with other cancer survivors."

Stephanie participates in lung cancer walks. She also goes to international meetings, where she networks with other lung cancer survivors. She shared her experience with this:

> That, for me, was a huge help. There were a bunch of different topics that were discussed, and then other survivors shared their stories, what they've been through, and again, just gave a lot of hope, especially for those of us there who were relatively newly diagnosed.

Stephanie does advocacy work because she wants to network and meet other survivors. Together, she and her fellow survivors can discuss different topics and share stories. She values hearing stories because they give her hope. So in Stephanie's experience, connecting with other survivors gives hope. That is why she pursues as many advocacy opportunities as she can.

In advocacy, some participants found opportunities for some positive experiences. This is what Sharon described. She said, "I've been able to take advantage of lots of opportunities to find some positivity in the diagnosis." Sharon travels to lung cancer summits in different cities all over. She went to one in Washington, DC, and described the importance of the trip:

> I was able to travel to separate events in Washington, DC, this year to meet with lawmakers to try to get increased attention and research funding for lung cancer.

When I interviewed Sharon, she had just returned from the International Association of the Study of Lung Cancer Conference in Toronto.

> I've tried to reach out and find every opportunity that I can to not just gain information for myself but also for the other advocates for this disease and for the survivors. That was an incredible experience just because of the other survivors we met.

Some of these opportunities offer a scholarship for survivors, which helps. Her husband was also able to meet other husband caregivers, just like himself. She also attended a Lung Cancer Alliance Summit, where she talked with congressional members about lung cancer and funding. She described,

> That was an incredible experience and completely different from other summits I've been to because it was more focused on political action.

She was also able to meet with senators and representatives from the State of Wisconsin to talk about the upcoming passage of a bill that would provide additional funding for lung cancer research. For Sharon, political activism is never separate from the experience of living with cancer.

In a slightly different vein, sharing the experiences and feelings with others is what Cynthia found meaningful. She explained,

> I became pretty much determined that I was going to throw myself into as much advocacy work as possible for bringing awareness to lung cancer doing fundraising for lung cancer events, and serving as an advocate for the cancer community.

Specifically, she described this as her coping strategy:

> That's been a huge coping strategy for me. The more involved and educated I become, the more connections that I make in that community and the more hopeful I feel for myself and the patients who are going to come after me.

Her advocacy work focused on bringing awareness and raising funds. For Cynthia, what was most important was sharing experiences and feelings with other survivors. Advocacy also allowed her to reshape her identity and to feel in control of who she is. Now, she is not only a patient; she is also an advocate. Advocacy can be more than simply an individual coping strategy. For Cynthia, the more she knows, the more she is able to help others. It is a coping strategy for the collective.

Advocacy has also helped some of the participants to restore an image they prided themselves in having. Amy explained,

> I've done a few things in my life that other people thought were fearless. It naturally just evolved in me wanting to do advocacy work, knowing that I have some gifts to share. I also have the knowledge base that people who are newly diagnosed generally do not have. I can be not only their adviser and their support system but also their defender if need be, and everybody needs that when they're going through this. There isn't enough of it.

While Amy receives care in a prestigious hospital, she recognizes that patient support and social services are not up to standards. She thinks health care providers are "overworked; they're hurried." Amy feels she has a presence that makes people feel very comfortable with her, and "they tend to talk easily about their problems." She has a gift, and sharing her gift is essential to her.

She realizes from being around other patients and being a patient herself that newly diagnosed patients do not have enough knowledge about the illness. That is why cancer survivors need defenders. For her, sharing about her experiences and what she has learned is also rebuilding and restoring an identity for her that had been threatened by cancer.

That is why taking the initiative to raise awareness and advocate for better care for lung cancer patients is what some patients choose to do. Katherine explained that it "became one of the biggest outlets for me."

Shortly after her diagnosis, one of her friends reached out to her to ask, "What do you think about organizing a race to raise some money for research?" They started planning for a 5K race, which took place a few months later. Katherine shared with pride that they had over 300 runners.

For her, that kind of planning and preparation was "a hugely positive outlet." It changed how Katherine viewed herself:

> So instead of sitting and mourning about what's going to come next, when will the medication stop working, and will there be another option for me, what I'm doing is finding a way to raise money to give to researchers to try to help make those options available. So that helps me.

For Katherine and others like her, advocacy is a positive outlet that prevents them from passively sitting and mourning their fate. It helps them. Katherine and others are aware that when they decide to go out and advocate, they are also finding meaning for their own experience. This isn't anyone claiming to be a hero but rather is the realization that the person is also serving oneself by serving others.

However, advocacy cannot be the only strategy used. Being on the go and exposed to other people's suffering can deprive the person of their reserves of energy and well-being. Justin alluded to this when he spoke about his advocacy. He noted first that "for me to advocate and to help others who are experiencing this type of cancer or any kind of cancer is somehow bringing down my levels of anxiety," but because he is active in the community, he has also come across a few people who were not doing well. He noted that encounters with those people who were having difficulties and had no real medical options left were "increasing my level of anxiety." Justin is taking advantage of counseling that is offered by the organization he works for as part of the job's benefits, and he has an appointment to talk with a counselor about that. He went on to say,

> I'm struggling to help on one side, which has helped me handle and cope with my condition by listening to other people who are going through it, and I'm not the only one experiencing this. It's not like misery loves company but to understand another person and to show them what I've been through and to give them hope also gives me hope.

Justin tries to manage his anxieties by doing more physical activity as much as he can, "which means trying to go for a walk." For him, advocacy and helping others is helping himself. At the same time, hearing other people's stories can be hard, and other strategies to support one's resilience are needed. Exercising and talking to a therapist can come to provide more endurance.

Sometimes, you can have a need to find other places to restore a sense of well-being and to rest.

Volunteering

Many participants who have talents that are relevant to their peers and community started volunteering. James, for example, dedicates a significant part of his time to nonprofit work. He explains,

> I am doing what I like doing. Helping others in the support group is something I get pleasure from. I do quite a lot of work with a variety of different nonprofit organizations, and that gives me the value in my life.

His work in nonprofit gives him a sense of value and purpose because it is good. He also draws pleasure from doing this kind of work. It is not dissimilar to what he did all his life in caring for and serving others. It is like work in terms of what it brings in meaning and value. The recognition is not material, and the compensation is not in money; instead, his work helps other cancer survivors. He explains,

> I have been spending a lot of time now helping the online support group, where I spend hours every day reading posts and answering people's questions. I'm also very involved with the management of the group. It's my new job. I've helped patients all my life as a dentist, and now I'm helping a different type of patient. It's still part of being a doctor; I'm just doing it differently.

James is aware that it is his coping strategy as well. Helping others is part of who he is. It is part of continuing to be a doctor and continuing to do the work he values. In volunteer work, there is the win-win that you may be also helping yourself while you are helping someone else. The two are intertwined in harmony. People who volunteer their time and talents value the opportunity and privilege to volunteer.

People with experience in management and organization also volunteer those skills. Richard explained,

> Once I learned that the medication was working, I still needed to do something productive toward cancer that was focused on feeling hope.

He first volunteered for a conference call that some of the group members asked for, and that call led to another call that led into a twenty-plus member outreach management team that wanted to get serious with structuring all their research and advocacy efforts. But Richard is just as engaged as ever, saying, "I don't see it stopping. As long as they'll have me help, I will help."

Doing volunteering work helps others and brings hope to the volunteer. As they participate in more volunteer activities and see in the eyes of those they are helping the impact of their work, some participants hoped that more people would volunteer. Amanda spoke about the spreading impact of her volunteer work:

> I became a volunteer at our cancer hospital and our lung cancer screening clinic every other Monday afternoon. I also helped interview Ohio State students who wanted to volunteer at our cancer hospital. I volunteered to serve coffee and refreshments to caretakers during Caretakers' Month. I've volunteered at our skin cancer screening; I've volunteered at three of those. I have visited my lung cancer doctor's lab a couple of times, and my granddaughter, who is nineteen and a freshman in college, ended up volunteering at my lung cancer doctor's lab all summer.

Amanda reflected how her involvements in all these activities was the result of a far-reaching and exciting series of events that she "would never have anticipated participating in before having lung cancer." She feels that

> It's because I have the energy and a little bit of knowledge, I can help people understand what's going on with lung cancer and lung cancer research, and encourage people to donate money to fund education and research to hopefully take away some of the stigma surrounding lung cancer.

She was frustrated that many people think lung cancer is a disease you cause yourself to contract. "The first question a lot of people asked me was, 'Were you a smoker?' And I often reply, "Anyone with lungs can get lung cancer." In reflecting again on her volunteer work, Amanda added,

> I feel like I'm giving back because I can and because I want to. I'm hopeful other people will catch this volunteering disease and stop playing cards in the afternoon and give some time to more worthwhile causes.

The notion of giving back to the community is salient. There is also the desire that people will volunteer more because volunteering is good. One can argue that the lived experience of a lung cancer patient will be qualitatively different if everyone volunteered a little more for the betterment of the whole group.

These cancer patients also chose to spend their time doing what is meaningful to them and found space to do that while volunteering their work. That is a position that John shares. He summed it up with, "I'm trying to do things that are meaningful to me."

Before his diagnosis, he had started a business that gives people tools to prep their meals. When he developed cancer, he turned that business into "kind of like a nonprofit." He explained, "I do my meal plan still, but I offer them for free to cancer patients." He sends out meal plans with recipes and a shopping list that cancer patients can use to help them with their nutrition. He remarked,

> That's meaningful to me because I feel like I'm helping people in the same situation, so I think that also helps me live with purpose and have some meaning.

He contributes his talents to nonprofit work as well. By turning his business into a nonprofit organization, he now volunteers in his capacity to help others, and that makes him live with purpose and have meaning, which is good. For him, it is essential to do things that are meaningful as it helps him live with purpose.

Mentoring

Cancer survivors not only have the talents they brought from their lives before the diagnosis to the experience of the illness, they also develop new ones by being ill. The lived experience of a patient is the principal teacher. They learn from being a patient, and they value what they can then give to others. Some of them called it mentorship.

Becoming a mentor is how Rebecca explained how her coping strategy evolved. She became involved in a support group where she first exchanges an email with someone seeking help, and then she meets and talks to the person one-on-one. These are individuals with the same type of diagnosis that she has. She noted that "they go through very similar things." She was once the mentee, and she remembers how she reached out to ask her adviser for advice when her medicine started giving her rashes. She notes, "I could talk to somebody, and she'd say, 'Well, I've tried this. Well, I've tried that,' or 'Ask your doctor about this.'" She appreciated having someone who knew what she was going through, so later, she became a mentor herself.

> I've always been a researcher where I research stuff. Even like for a vacation. I research where to stay, what to do, and then I like to share that information with people. And this became the same part of my life and kept my mind activated.

She can now share what she has learned with somebody else, which she enjoys.

> When they have different questions, I can be, "Oh! Yes, I went through that," or "I felt that way, too." And it's still positive to relive some of that and to share my experiences.

Being a mentor also allowed Rebecca to reflect on her own experience:

> It taught me how much I kind of lived in a nonactive way at the beginning. But I like to be active and talk about it and be involved. It just gives me life and hope.

Mentoring is now a primary coping strategy for Rebecca:

> So, to talk about it and to process through, I think it helps me cope with all that. It helped me sharing with somebody else and having someone else understand.

Many participants found through their experience that it is good to share and to talk to those who have also gone through the same. The person learns from others with similar conditions. Furthermore, hope can be gleaned from participating in these conversations.

I realize that some may worry about what is being shared not being the result of a systematic inquiry, and that is a legitimate concern. Many participants, however, found it of the utmost value to them to connect with others and learn from one another.

Other participants are also finding purpose in mentoring. Stephanie got a pen pal through an online forum, and she also met someone who has lung cancer with a similar mutation as hers (EGFR). She emailed the person and got to talk to them more, which was very meaningful to her. She said,

> That seemed to give my life a whole different meaning and purpose. I said to myself, "Oh, gosh! Maybe this is my purpose now. Maybe I can help others and be involved in that aspect."

After that, Stephanie started researching more and preparing to go back to work. She explained that she "felt like I was strong enough, and I love to keep my mind active." She also continued her school work:

> When I was diagnosed, I was probably six or seven classes from getting my Master of Science in nursing (MSN). So during the year that I was off work, I continued with my classes and got my MSN. And that helps me keep my mind active, too.

As she continued to learn more and search for information, people who had just been diagnosed with cancer started to reach out to her. She shared, "I become their advocate to say reach out, ask questions, be involved." For her, the bottom line was that "the biggest thing I've learned is keeping my mind active by helping these advocates."

Having someone to mentor and exchange thoughts with can give life a purpose and meaning, and purpose is essential.

Participating in Research

Another coping strategy that exemplifies being mindful of others and paying it forward to the community is participation in research studies.

Taking part in studies is how Stephanie explains her coping strategy,

> I have participated in studies from the very beginning, on diagnosis, I had part of the brain tumor sent for further testing. I want to help somebody else, and hopefully, one day, I think every cancer survivor's dream, there will be a cure. So I feel that by sharing my story, I can hopefully help someone

else and also let them realize that there is hope and it's not a death sentence, like so many of us are told.

Even in the study that led to this book, by sharing their stories, these participants are motivated by a desire to help others. They have learned that lung cancer is not a death sentence. However, this realization did not come to them immediately. It took labor and struggle. So, if they can make it easier for others by giving them hope and making the journey more tolerable, they will do so.

One can also find in this a desire to affirm that realization, that it is not a death sentence, and in receiving the recognition, one also gains more certainty.

We all need this recognition in order to trust that what we believe in is true. Finding that our conception of the experience is valid and comparable to others gives us better certainty.

Holding onto Relationships

For some, coping came through relationships and in connecting with family, friends, and support groups. Some also resorted to finding a therapist. Others found love and care with their animals.

Family

Family appears here again not only as a source of meaning but as a means of support in day-to-day life. Engaging with family is a way to cope with the illness. Some participants described spending time with family and having regular phone calls to be their coping strategy. For example, Kim shared,

> I have a very supportive family, so I do spend time with them.
> We have frequent phone calls.

She has one brother who lives overseas. They are "in more communication now than we ever have been in the past." Her kids are also home from college. One of them is home because she is done with college and the other one is home for the summer. Kim said, "At least right now all four of us are together, so yes, that's just very helpful." Kim copes by leveraging the support of her family.

A supportive family makes a difference, and that is good. Kim, like others in similar situations, appreciates and enjoys her family's support. Staying in touch with supportive family is, for some participants, the main coping strategy.

Others also cope by being involved with family and doing things with them. Amanda remarked,

> I prepare our meals at home. I run a lot of errands. I spend time with my family. I attend my grandchildren's sporting events. I have a granddaughter who's in the choir, and she's in a high school musical. She used to play volleyball. I try to go to most of their games and activities when I can.

For Amanda and those like her, being involved with family, spending time with them and doing family activities, is part of who they are. Being involved with family is how they cope.

Friends

Friends are an important source of support. Friends come or are sought out to support the person's coping. Simply talking to friends helps, as James explained,

> Just the fact that I have shared it with others all along is my form of therapy; talking about it with friends is a form of therapy.

For many people, simply talking to friends is therapeutic. With the illness, some participants worked to restore their social relationships because they found them to be essential. Robert reflected on this:

> I went back out into my social group and came out to them and repaired some connections. I'm going out and hanging out as I used to, and it feels good. I'm just psychologically trying to put myself in homeostasis similar to how I used to be, but more positively. So, I'm hanging out with people, informing them about my cancer but also not letting that monopolize our conversations. Not that I wanted to hide it around them at all because they all know about it and they've all come to me, but I also want to show them that this is different—this is what I look like, and this is how I am, as a lung cancer patient.

Robert is rebuilding his relationships with friends. He wants the balance he used to have with these relationships and hopes to achieve that by telling them about his cancer without letting it monopolize the conversation.

For Robert, it was a choice to go back to social groups. It is a choice to repair relationships broken by whatever takes place in life. For Robert and other people with cancer, it is most important that they can choose where to prioritize cancer in these relationships. Robert wanted to share, yet he was mindful of others, and he valued these relationships and doing things in moderation, including drinking with old friends. He realizes that he now has to watch himself better, and he constantly strives for homeostasis.

Robert is a lung cancer patient but not *only* a lung cancer patient. He is authentic, mindful, and aware of the values of others and the meaning in being around them.

People also used a variety of strategies to keep their friends involved and updated. Ashley told of her solution:

> I've made a lot of connections with friends and family. I set
> up a web page on my cancer, mylifeline.org, so that I can keep
> people updated.

She wants to keep her family and friends updated because they want to be updated. It is not just about listening and talking. Here, the mode of interaction is in one direction, but that works because other people care to know.

At times, however, interactions with others, such as colleagues and acquaintances, can be awkward. The person grappling with cancer is in a particular state of mind and grappling with existential matters. At times, it is harder for them to relate to other people's day-to-day trivial matters. It can likewise be harder for other people to connect to the person's struggle and, at times, say the right thing. Emily gave an example:

> There are those irritating interpersonal interactions. There is
> your colleague who comes in and cries about his mother who
> died of cancer. Then he goes on and self-indulges about how
> he can't believe you are not taking medical leave because he
> would take a leave so he could write his poetry. And, I'm like,
> don't you understand that I'm just trying to be alive?

When people come to talk to her and share things about themselves, she often becomes troubled by what they say.

> Everywhere you go, people are telling you the most
> unbelievable stuff about themselves. People you don't know,

and it's kind of funny. People either run up to me and tell me about everybody that they know who died in a horrible way or people who were supposed to die but they didn't die because they ate cherries or apricots, or how they're worried about themselves because their uncle died of something.

Talking to people can become harder when they don't quite understand. At times, it can appear as if people worry about themselves when they hear cancer stories, and that becomes their whole focus. Sometimes, they awkwardly tell the person who is struggling things that can never help. People are not always thoughtful enough to avoid self-indulgence. They don't realize that bringing stories of death to someone grappling with death is not kind. They also sometimes do not understand that the person probably has thought about the practical matters, and they don't need unsolicited advice.

Let's call it out. When people hear about cancer in someone who is like themselves in the sense of being the same age or having a similar lifestyle, they can sometimes look inwardly and worry more about themselves than anything else. While this is a natural reaction, it is also incredibly insensitive.

Cancer patients are just trying to stay alive, and it can be tempting to ask those insensitive people to leave us alone if all they have to say are ruminations about trivialities.

Still, to be fair, we are all awkward beings and don't always know what to say to someone living with cancer. It isn't easy, for many people, to understand how the other person feels, especially at difficult times, like when dealing with cancer.

Cancer patients may find themselves deciding to be selective in their relationships. As they struggle with insensitivity, some participants had to avoid what they described as negative relationships. Other people often do not quite understand the priorities of cancer patients, and as a result, they say things that are not courteous.

Mary shared about "a woman that I knew from baseball who was very judgmental." Mary described this woman as someone who "always seems to find the negative of things." One time, the lady said something to Mary that was not right, and it was at the time when Mary was dealing with the new diagnosis of a brain mass. The comment was insensitive, and Mary had to make a decision.

> I just decided and said that time, "You know, I'm not going to deal with this person anymore." I blocked her from my social media. I blocked her from the phone. I let other people around me know that I was not going to allow this person to be a part of my life.

Mary went on to give more background about the incident, explaining,

> I used to run the concession stand. She had taken over the concession stand that year when I was no longer able to do it. I also just wanted to be able to spend more time enjoying my son's games than being in the concession stand. At one of these games, and it was the same week that I was diagnosed with the brain mass, I wasn't feeling well. I wasn't able to stay through the whole game. I started to get up to leave, and she commented, "Well, if you're going to get up and leave, you think you can go to the concession stand and clean it for me?"

It was troubling to Mary that the person would not understand. To her, it sounded as if the woman was saying, "You're leaving your child's game to go home and go to bed? Why don't you go over and clean the concession stand for me instead, then."

Mary didn't appreciate it. She blocks those she describes as "negative people" from her life, and she doesn't have remorse for that. It is a perfectly understandable option for many people who struggle to be understood. They prioritize what matters most to them.

Because of these concerns about how others would treat or mistreat them, and because of concerns for privacy, participants grappled with announcing their illness or with keeping it private.

In the camp that was pro-sharing, Andrew explained,

> What made a difference, believe me, I had my low days, is the connection. I had a lot of friends who reached out. I

announced on Facebook, finally. I tend to be a private person. I don't wear my heart on my sleeve, but I announced as part of November's lung cancer awareness month that I had lung cancer Stage 4 and that's how people have known. I got such great feedback. A lot of friends came out of the woodwork. I probably had people reaching out once a day. I found that connection with people, just the mere human bond that you get from reconnecting, made a huge difference in my day. The day that didn't include any connection wasn't nearly as easy to deal with. So I had decided, despite my introversion and my tendency to spend my time in my head, that human connection is one of the best things that life is all about, and I'm going to make sure that I keep it up.

There is meaning in sharing, and there is a purpose as well.

People don't share their diagnosis just for themselves, however, but also do so for the sake of others. For Andrew, the motivation was raising awareness. Sharing about the diagnosis is an attempt to make people more aware. This was also the motive for Kim, who explained,

> I've also found that since my diagnosis, I've been able to reconnect with people that I had not been in touch with for a long time. I know everyone is different about sharing their news with others, but when I was first diagnosed, I wanted to tell everybody I knew that I had just been diagnosed. I didn't want to keep any of it a secret or any of it private. I wanted as many people as possible to know so that, first of all, they would be aware that, hey, even if you're a nonsmoker, you can get lung cancer. I also wanted more people praying for me because most of the other people I know are also Catholic. So, I figured the more people praying for me, the better.

For some, more important than sharing with the public is sharing with cancer survivors. That was Cynthia's position:

> It was helpful, but I felt like what would be more important

to me was sharing experiences and feelings with other cancer patients. So I joined several online communities through Facebook and met so many cancer patients that way.

Likewise, Cynthia feels that sharing with those who live the same experience is more relevant and helpful. This position comes in addition to the desire to normalize the experience and to reach a broader audience to converse with and tell others that their struggle is not solely their own but that others could also experience it.

Participants in the other camp decided to be private. Mary explained her reasoning:

> We are more like a private family; you don't reach out a whole lot to others. I don't like being asked how I feel, and "You still feel OK?" or "How are you doing?"

Mary didn't like people asking how she was feeling, and it is true that not everyone likes to be asked that. People should not assume that everyone wants to be asked how they are doing and should take their cues from the individual. Some people are private, and they wish to not be bothered.

Others worried that announcing may be perceived as a desire for sympathy, and they didn't want to be in a position of receiving pity. Jessica shared her thoughts on this:

> I'm a private person. I am not advertising that I have cancer, and a lot of people don't know I do and won't unless there's a need that comes up. I'm not hiding it, but there's only a handful of coworkers that I've told. I've been told a lot of times, and I know you've heard this before too, that we don't look sick, you know, no one would ever know we have it. I don't dwell on the fact that I have cancer, and there are times when I forget it until someone, you know, sends me something or I have to go for an appointment or whatever. I don't get up every day and say, "I can't do this; I have cancer."

Jessica is cautious about how the subject of her illness is raised. This position comes up in Jessica's family interactions:

> It's a joke in my family about pulling the cancer card. You
> know, when you pull the cancer card, "Hey, I got cancer, you
> need to be nicer to me." I think that there are people out there,
> and maybe they're doing it under the guise of education, but I
> believe there are people out there who probably advertise the
> fact that they have cancer for the sympathy side of it. Maybe.
> I don't know. There are people out there who don't have a
> problem with showing that they have cancer because they can
> get a parking space up front. You know, disabled parking. I
> probably could get disability right now; I could probably get
> a handicapped sticker if I wanted to, but I'm not going to do
> that. As long as I'm able to walk across the parking lot, I'm
> going to do that, and I'm not going to take up a parking space
> for somebody who really needs it. I don't think I need it. I can
> walk across the parking lot.

For Jessica, cancer should not be waved around like a winning card.
She doesn't dwell on it. She would not advertise it and would not seek the
benefits others in her position might look for, such as parking permits for the
disabled. For her, it is crucial to not be mistaken as someone who advertises
their struggle to garner sympathy.

Some of the participants went so far as not telling members of their own
family about their illness. Christine shared,

> I decided not to tell the majority of people, so my children
> don't know. But I have a few friends who know. My husband
> and my parents know, as well. Nobody else knows. So, I really
> needed to talk to somebody about it.

For Christine, people do not need to know. However, a consequence
of her choice is that she did not have many people to talk to when she
needed someone.

Support Groups

Support groups were described by many as their primary coping strategy. They were lifesavers for some. Mary, for example, found a support group through someone who knows someone else who has a family member with illness. She explained what the online support group meant to her:

> It's about a lifesaver, just to be able to interact with people who have the same thing, who are going through the same journey and being able to know that if you put something out there, you're not going to be judged on what you're talking about and what you're questioning. There is also the expertise of all the different doctors people are seeing and in finding out what they are doing. And just the calm that I have in knowing that there are doctors out there dedicating their lives to helping us make this a manageable, chronic disease.

Being part of the group helped Mary change her perception of her illness, and she explained, "I'm finally to the point where I feel like I'm going to live for a while." For Mary, seeing other survivors live and thrive gave her some certainty that she will also be all right. Living examples do give assurance.

Susan had a similar experience. She was referred to join the group by her doctor, and Susan felt like the group gave her hope:

> Well, I would definitely say the online support group made a huge impact. The doctor at the cancer center is actually the one who told me about the group.
>
> I can see people who have had this diagnosis for ten-plus years compared to, you know, when I google prognosis for cancer that has spread to your brain and your liver, and it's telling me an average of eight months. So seeing long-term survivors was good.

For her, the group made an impact and gave her hope because she got to see people who had survived many years with the same type of cancer as hers. She thought, "Other people fared well, so why wouldn't I, too?" People join the support groups and find not only help but also friendship. Elizabeth told how she met other survivors through support groups and then connected again at advocacy events, and since then, they have maintained a strong bond:

> It gives me much hope that I have met so many young lung cancer survivors just like me. I have maintained friendships long-distance through Facebook.

Those who are local to her she gets together with or takes walks with as they "share life's moments and pieces, and so that's been helpful."

For some of the others, these groups are primarily sources of helpful information. That is what Jessica described:

> I stayed off the internet because that was scaring me to death. I pretty much stayed off of Facebook because I couldn't handle seeing people complaining about a headache; that was bothering me. They were just too painful. I removed myself from Facebook, but then I found the online support on Facebook. For some reason, I've seen that as my major coping mechanism. I don't post much there, but I read it, and for me, that's my coping.

Jessica realized from seeing other individuals in the group that although she has cancer, she is fortunate. She noted, "I'm still able to work; I'm still able to do. My life has not changed that much with this diagnosis, not like some other people in my group." She also reflects on her privileges:

> There are people from all over the world who are in the group, and I'm realizing now how fortunate I am that I'm in the United States and have great insurance. Some people can't even get the drug, and if they do, they have to pay a lot for it. They have huge out-of-pocket costs. I have to pay, but not anything like some people do. For me, it's made me realize that I'm very, very lucky compared to some people.

Jessica also realized that some people are faring quite well and "even have it better than I do." She believes those are the patients who are getting "no evidence of disease" (NED) on their scans. She added, "They told me I would never hear those words of NED."

We cannot, at times, help but compare ourselves to others. If others are faring well and we are not, we feel sad. Is this another form of our human jealousy?

For some participants, the support groups have helped them regain a sense of purpose they had lost with their illness. Nancy is among them, and reflected,

> I can't believe I didn't mention that. That group has been the biggest healing for me. The biggest turning point for me was joining that group and reaching out to other people and hearing their experiences that were so similar to mine. They had the same sadness. They had the same anger, and it brought me out of my deep grief because I got to help other people.

Nancy would spend hours "every single day" when she first joined. "Hours and hours and hours, commenting on people's posts and giving them support, checking in with them." She still does that and has befriended patients and their caregivers who are her age, and she checks in with them. She explains,

> It gives me a purpose and a meaning to be able to help them get through this.

It gave her purpose and meaning: by helping others, the person helps themselves. And she wanted to help others.

People were not entangled in the questions, am I helping others to help myself? They did it because it is meaningful, and in it, there is a purpose.

There is reconstructing of a role and reconnecting with an identity that was challenged with the illness.

The important things regarding these groups, however, is the understanding that she gets from talking and listening to people. This is what Michael said,

The Facebook page is a great place to go. First of all, it's filled with a bunch of people who almost have the same story as mine. We landed in the same spot, so we all understand our feelings at times.

Michael finds the information there particularly helpful. He explains,

It almost seems like whatever instance that someone, wherever scenario someone lands into, that someone got an answer for you or a solid recommendation on what your next step should be.

On the group, people with multiple stories land in the same spot, and they understand each other's feelings and experiences.

And it is good to be understood.

The information available in these groups is also appreciated, as Ashley explains,

Connecting with these people, and they come from all walks of life that I find that there are many people in there who are medical professionals and researchers.

The information available to her made her also compare her experience with other people who have the same path. She shares an example,

Reading posts once made me wonder, why they haven't done a scan since I started with the oncologist.

That gave her a question to ask the oncologist at her next visit. She also finds the group to consist of positive people. She explains,

They are very supportive. If somebody's having a good day or a bad day at either end of that spectrum, they're there with words of encouragement, and it's a positive connection for me.

There is a wealth of information and experiences, and these are especially important for those who have only a few friends or family to support or have little capacity to get out to get the support in person. The group allows the cancer patient to connect with people.

Besides the online support groups, some individuals joined in-person groups. Here is Donna who joined a cancer support group. The group consisted of young adult cancer survivors, and they meet once a month in a support group setting. They also did social activities. For Donna, it was helpful and comforting to be around some other people at the same stage in life with her.

The groups usually have ten to fifteen people at each meeting. They are an hour long, and everybody sits in a circle. There's a couple of couches and then some chairs, and there's a facilitator who is a social worker and a cancer survivor as well. Donna describes,

> The facilitator is really kind. She has everybody at the beginning go around and introduce themselves; there's always somebody new in the room. You can talk about what kind of cancer you have and when you were diagnosed, and what's going on in your life or if there's any topic that you'd like to talk about.

Donna enjoys the experience. She shared a reflection,

> I like to listen to what other people are going through, more than talking about myself. Because to me, listening to what other people are doing is helpful, so I don't feel alone in this and so that I can learn from what they've done as well. I have also shared about my own experiences, and people have suggestions, "Hey, did you ever think of this?" Or, "Oh my gosh, I know how you feel because I've been through that as well." It just makes you feel like you are part of the group and a community that nobody wants to be part of, but you are not alone in it. It's just the perfect setting to make sense of things.

In these groups, some of the participants found recognition and understanding. For some participants, it is the relationships that matter the most. Richard elaborated,

Relationships matter most, and the relationship that I started developing with many of the cancer community members fueled me to really get involved to do the advocacy and research, to do my part in fundraising so that we can get more research grants. There are special bonds with these people because they are like-minded, and they want to do the same thing. It created a new family for me.

He considers the smaller management team he's working with on the support group to be his family and explains, "I consider them as support for me, so I give them the same." He also enjoys the work he is contributing:

I like to pull myself into things I am highly interested in. It became something to figure out and invest my time in, with learning more about the science behind cancer and the treatments coming down the road, what it means with all these lung cancer organizations in the space, who is doing what and accomplishing what and how with all these programs that are coming together, are they helping or hurting. I have a curious mind, and I wanted to learn a whole new industry. I'm dealing with lung cancer as a new industry.

For some participants, the support group gave positivity and tools. Carol shared about her experience. The support group she joined went on for twelve weeks, and she met other people who happened to all be women, all with different types of cancers. Carol noted, "That was really helpful. They gave us a lot of tools and a lot of ways to shift our mind-set around."

She learned relaxation techniques, which was also helpful to her. Carol tries to surround herself with "positive people." That is why she appreciated the support group, because they understand her. She remarked,

It was so nice to be in the same room where you get to explain yourself, and people understood. There was real positive energy. That kind of thing just lifts you up. It just kind of nourishes the soul.

There is also the notion that shifting one's mind-set is possible, that the person can, in the right place and with the right tools, turn their frame of reference around. This agency is good, Carol would argue. Focusing on positivity is useful, and avoiding what is negative is good. One may be concerned with this aversion to the negative yet still be understanding of why someone with such an illness would want to find positivity here and there.

Melissa brings attention to a nuanced notion in the experience of patients in regard to how we react to other people's suffering. In the beginning, she went to a cancer support community and joined a group. There, she made friends and found a lot of help. They had activities together. She was thankful as she came closer to seeing others' suffering. Melissa described her experience: "The smartest thing I could have done. Nicest group of people. We are friends to this day, and that was in 2013. So, five years ago, and we're still friends."

They still get together, and the group is supportive of one another even though all of them have graduated from the group. The group also gave her support despite not being lung cancer specific; it was for all different kinds of cancer. She says, "We understood each other. We cared about each other." She continued,

> I think hearing other people's concerns and worries, some of them made you feel better. So many people were bankrupt and horrible things had happened. And I had good insurance, and I was grateful for that. But then, so many issues that we found were similar and that we all still had lives and the kids or husbands or this or that. We all still had all of life's regular problems and issues as well as cancer issues.

She does believe the group members helped each other, and they relied on each other. They even met outside the group, especially whenever there was a crisis or a celebration. She shares,

> If there were a birthday we would meet outside the group. Also, once all of us graduated, a lot of people finished their chemo and were not on therapy anymore, and a lot of people had to go back to work.

They also met for fundraisers for the cancer support community. Melissa reflected on the beauty and sadness of this group,

> It's a wonderful group of educated, intelligent women. We had a few guys who we loved in the group. They all died. That is the downside of all these support groups is that the people keep dying. And the upside of it is that we are the ones who understand what you are going through.

Not everyone gets it other than those friends who have a similar illness. For Melissa, we feel better when we hear other people's misery as we become aware that our conditions are not the worst. We become grateful that we're not the ones who are in that deep struggle.

For some, joining these support groups can be described as the best thing to happen. Andrew is also a member of a group that includes patients with the same mutation he has. There is one person who has survived almost five years. Another one is now an eight-year survivor. There's a ten-year survivor as well. For Andrew,

> There isn't anything better in life than to go to a group of people who are surviving with the same thing you have and will understand you and listen to you and give you hope.

Andrew tries to never miss opportunities to get together with those people. He argues that being in a survivor group should be part of every person's treatment plan and explains,

> If you want to have hope, go meet with somebody who's survived your disease for a long time. Then, those statistics just look like statistics. You've got a warm body in front of you who can tell you "It's going to be OK. You can do this." God knows how much difference that's made.

Connecting with survivor groups is one of the best things we can do. Because if you want hope, you should meet survivors. Andrew pointed out that survivor groups should be part of any person's treatment plan. It is almost universally good.

Survivors understand.

Therapy

Some participants recognize the importance and value of engaging in therapy to cope. Emily explained,

> I knew that therapy was a good idea right away. I think that there's a place for having someone I can talk to outside of the family. I don't need a lot of insight, like I'm not looking for a life-transforming insight kind of thing, but I am hoping for someone who has compassion and has a good sense of humor who can help me. There are irritating interpersonal interactions that are hard to manage, and there's grief.

Making time for therapy can be hard. And seeking a therapist is, for many, not about getting transformational insights. But therapy is a vital help. Compassion is needed, and maybe a sense of humor.

Some participants asked their doctor about seeing someone to talk to, and those who have a good fit with their therapist have developed a better understanding. Carol started to see a therapist and described therapy as very helpful. Her therapist recommended coping mechanisms and gave her books to read in addition to providing counseling that she thought would be most helpful. The therapist she found has been active in supporting the mental and emotional health of cancer patients, survivors, caregivers.

Carol dealt with anxiety, and her psychiatrist prescribed anxiety medications and also gave her a list of therapists' names. Still, it was hard for her to find one right away. She went to a few who all said, "I'm sorry; I'm full, but you might want to talk to these people." Then she went to those people and heard, "These people are full, but you might want to talk to these other people." Finally, she found somebody who actually had an opening in her schedule and was able to see Carol. Because of her work with the counselor, Carol felt she has a better understanding.

She explained, "It doesn't have to be a death sentence; you can try to live your life. There is so much development and research going on right now."

Her therapist has said, literally, that this is the best time to get cancer. "If I were to get cancer twenty years ago, I wouldn't be taking targeted therapy like one pill a day type of thing." Carol was able to share her fears and her anxieties, and that helped her cope. When she went to the first appointment, the counselor gave her a USB stick with all the guided relaxation and breathing techniques. She found them helpful and said, "I feel better when I do it. I try to do it at least a few minutes a day."

They talked about her fears and worries, and she received helpful exercises. It was notable that the therapist had worked before with cancer patients and had experience. It is often not easy to find a therapist who has availability and expertise. Carol felt better, and the strategies used by her therapist were helpful.

With the therapist, Carol learned communication techniques, especially with regard to talking to her husband. The cancer diagnosis was "emotionally devastating" to her. But she felt as if, to him, it was, "at least you should feel lucky to be alive." It was as if he were saying that she should be more positive, and she felt they weren't matching very well at that time.

The therapist gave her techniques for how to help him understand how she feels. Her husband would say things that weren't exactly what she needed to hear, and to her, he didn't seem to understand her devastation. So now she is learning communication techniques to use when people say insensitive things to her.

What can be devastating to one person may be considered not even relevant by others.

Finding ways to reconcile the different positions is essential, especially for couples. Finding ways to reexamine what is judged to be relevant or trivial is just as important.

Therapeutic relationships evolve over time as the person's position in relation to cancer changes. And cancer does not always stay the focus of the conversation. This is what Sharon found. She continued to see her therapist, and they had a tremendous therapeutic rapport. She noted, "That's just incredibly rewarding for me." This therapeutic relationship was helpful for Sharon in several ways. She explained:

> At the beginning of our therapeutic relationship, we talked about lung cancer only. But then it evolved to the point that I can speak with her about the normal stressors in my life as a mom, a daughter, a wife, a career person.

Using cognitive behavioral therapy, Sharon's therapist is helping her reframe how she thinks and does certain things. She is becoming able to look at her thoughts differently and examine them using other perspectives. She is also becoming more able to consider her emotions about things that have happened from a different perspective to increase her coping skills and to engage more meaningfully with people, especially her husband and other family members.

The therapist has helped with normal stressors and not just cancer, although the focus at first was primarily cancer. Now Sharon prides herself in being able to consider her emotions and see what is happening to her from a different perspective. It is as if there is only so much that the person can say about cancer, and then the topic evolves to other life matters.

At times, however, the struggle can be too challenging even for a therapist. That was Mary's experience. She struggled with depression and anxiety. Her doctor put her on medications for both and also suggested that she start seeing a therapist. Mary said,

> I went and saw a therapist, and I remembered crying throughout the whole thing. And this woman, she looks like a deer in the headlights. She had no idea what to do with me.

At that time, Mary was "fixating on the fact that I was going to die." She wished she had met someone who had the same thing she had or someone who could understand. It is not very helpful when the person you seek help from does not know how to help you. One might think that Mary may have been too deeply depressed and had too much anxiety to be a candidate for therapy.

Not everyone felt they needed counseling. For example, Larry did not think he needed it. He described his reasoning:

> My thinking about counselors is they explain rather simple

things to most people who don't understand simple things. I'm a pretty reflective person. I think about what has happened and what could happen, and I don't feel as though a counselor is going to add to that. And not to disparage this whole profession, I'm sure they help people all over the place, but I don't feel at all a need to be counseled.

Counseling may not be for everyone. For some, however, seeing a therapist is to help them stay resilient as they advocate for others. This is Justin's perspective:

I found that to handle the stress and to handle this diagnosis, for me to advocate and to help others who are experiencing this type of cancer or any kind of cancer, is somehow bringing down my levels of anxiety. Of late, though, I have found a few people who are not doing well, and that is increasing my level of anxiety. The organization I work for offers counseling as part of the benefits with the company, and I do have an appointment to talk with a counselor about that because I'm struggling with helping.

Helping others helps the person but can drain their reserve of energy and well-being. It is a struggle for some to be on the front lines supporting others, and it can be appealing and a comfort to recognize that there is not only one strategy that people use to cope.

Every strategy has scope or range and a limit. Advocacy helps the person by letting them realize purpose in helping others. However, it brings the challenge of being involved and occupied and exposed to struggle. Therapy then comes to open space for that person to exercise self-care and to accept being taken care of by others.

Some participants are using these complementing strategies: helping others and accepting help from others. One can think of the image of a circle of relief or a network of people holding hands to stay afloat—the person supports others and is in turn supported by others. One person cannot do it alone. For Justin, it is clear that advocacy and being around cancer survivors empowers and builds resilience.

But advocacy can overwhelm one person, and counseling can help.

Some who chose to keep their experience private brought similar reasoning in explaining seeing a therapist. Christine decided not to tell the majority of people, and even her children don't know. That, however, left her with few people to talk to. She really needed to talk to somebody about it and found counseling offered through the cancer center, then found a therapist on her own. Interestingly, however, she found herself almost teaching the therapist about her condition. The therapist learned from her about her cancer, and she learned from the therapist how to deal with it.

There are clearly many reasons to find a good therapist.

Animals

Some participants found help with coping in their pets. Debora was one who voiced this perspective:

> I walk the dogs, and I pet the cats. They take my mind off of
> my problems. They soothe and calm me. All animals do.

When I asked her to elaborate further, Debora laughed and explained,

> I don't know. I just love them because they are so cute. Some
> are very sweet. You know, the cats curl up, they're happy, and
> they like to be petted. And they make these calming sounds;
> it's nice. You forget your problems.

Animals can soothe and help. They can be therapeutic, and people can enjoy their company and find them calming. Some participants would go so far as recommending that those struggling with cancer get pets. They help as the person walks or spends time with them, and they can help take the person's mind off their problems.

Justin agreed that pets are therapeutic:

> We've never been, as a family, animal lovers. But we decided

to get a small dog because I learned that they could provide therapy to you when you have them around you or you're stroking them. So, I researched a breed that could help me do that. The dog, I must say, has been a tremendously positive thing because it does, in fact, bring calmness. It brings the stress levels down, plus I have an excuse to take the dog out for a walk and to get exercise.

Pets help with coping, especially if people are not around to give support. At times, pets are beneficial even when there are people around; some people may find their pets to be the best source of support. Samantha talked about her dogs:

I spend a lot of time with them. I take them for walks and talk to them and pet them.

The cat was not to be left out either.

And my cat, I do, too. Not go for a walk so much, but I talk to her a lot, and she sits on my lap and purrs.

Animals can be therapeutic support, and many participants expressed that they cope by spending time with their pets, giving and receiving affection and companionship.

Shifting Frameworks

People with cancer shift their frames of reference and their priorities. They choose, at times, to forget about their illness so they can carry on and deal with life affairs. Some try to be positive and few hold on to faith. Finally, some participants use humor to connect to others and stay in the mainstream of life.

Dealing with Practical Matters

Instead of being fixed on the struggle, some participants chose to focus on dealing with practical matters. Cynthia discussed this choice:

> Even right at the very beginning, friends and family were all praising my coping abilities, because although I do consider myself to be an emotional person, I was not falling apart and sobbing. I was initially extremely practical, and part of that I think is because during that hospitalization when they found that I have brain metastases, I was put on steroids. I was on fairly high doses of steroids, which probably helped my demeanor and attitude in those early days after the diagnoses because I was just extremely practical minded. I was not very emotional. At times I was, but for the most part, I thought OK, I have a serious illness. We need to deal with this very seriously. We are going to treat it very aggressively. But at the same time, I need a will. I need to make provisions for the care of my children. I need to take care of managing, getting all of my finances set up.

So Cynthia set up a trust and put all her assets into a trust for her kids. She also had a will drawn up and started going through things like all the family photos so that she could make sense of them and put together photo albums for her kids. She explained,

> I just kept thinking well, if I die in six months, I want to have

things a little more in shape than they are now, and I was very clear-minded about this was how I was going to get through coping. This was also right before Christmas when I was diagnosed, and we always have a huge beautiful Christmas, and I was determined to make that just the best ever because I thought this could potentially be my last.

While she identifies as an emotional person, Cynthia maintained her composure and focused on practical matters. She realized that being on steroids maybe had something to do with it, but regardless, her choice at first was to focus on practical issues such as finances, a will, setting up a trust, and putting together photo albums.

It is as if the patient senses an obligation; if they are dying soon, they should get things in shape to make it easier for their offspring. They needed to deal with it seriously, and they were first and foremost determined to get this vital work done. It seems to me that we humans pay attention to what we, and only we, can do. Those are our personal matters. But there is more to that.

Taking care of these affairs might also give you a sense of control and order at a time when both are disrupted.

Similarly, Larry shared thoughts about his wife and family.

The biggest impact is with my wife and her certainty about her future because she depends on me for some things. So we had to change her life a little bit in some ways. We moved to be closer to her work. So we had to sell a house or two along the way and find a place that could be good for her if I was not around. We stay close to family because family is going to be important for her in the future. We had a plan to probably move in with my son and his wife and daughter in the next six months, into a single house. So, we sell one more house, and we'll move in jointly.

Larry and his wife had to make changes in the family's living arrangements to adjust. Cancer makes people aware of the impact of this division in responsibility when suddenly accommodations need to be made to work around the absence of the person who used to do or take care of certain things. There is also this sense of wanting to make life easier for family.

This drive is essential for cancer patients.

People find themselves having to train their family to do the household and financial chores. Scott discussed this aspect:

> I had trained all the kids to do the yard work. One kid's in high school now. She does all the snow removal, the lawn care, and stuff.

While Scott looks normal to most people, his capacity for doing things like chores has declined. He needed to teach his kids to do the things he used to do to make sure family affairs are still manageable both with him still around, but in declining health, and after he is gone.

Scott and other patients in similar circumstances are acutely aware of their physical limitations and having to now rely on the kids to do chores. Their absence also means that others in the family, sometimes the children, must take over the responsibility for the household chores they used to deal with. That is not without cost. Scott describes how his daughter did the tax returns for the year prior, and there were mistakes. "I had to redo the whole thing, and we are still dealing with audits," he explained.

Having a sense of control and certainty becomes essential for some. To attain that, patients resort to making arrangements for after death. Planning the funeral, in the end, gives the ultimate sense of control and acceptance. Mary talked about this:

> When I was first diagnosed, I can remember being at work, and your mind is always, when you have idle times, constantly thinking about your final days. What are my kids going to do without me? And I could cry at the drop of a hat, and I was just breaking down emotionally, to the point where I would have to excuse myself. It got to the point where I felt like I was fixating on the end.

She was struggling and needed to do something. She continued,

> I needed to do things that I could have some control over.
> So I started planning my thoughts for my end regarding
> making my arrangements and estate planning, what I want
> my children to have, and what I want my extended family to
> have. I also planned what I want concerning a service or a
> funeral, whether it be cremation or casket or whatnot. I think
> it was probably about six months after diagnosis before I was
> finally able to sit down, and once I wrote everything out, I felt
> a lot better about it.

Mary only felt better once she had completed her planning, and that
gave her a sense of control, which helped. For Mary, she felt better once
she had accepted the end and was ready for it. Coming to terms with death
is not different from previous themes of reconciling with dying and not
being fearful of it. But here it takes a new shape. Whether here or there,
having a sense of solid feet on the ground and a sense of control is what the
participants desired, and you get that by reconciling with death and making
your arrangements.

Not thinking about it

For some participants, help was found in merely not thinking about the
struggle and not dwelling on it. Jessica tended to use this tactic and pointed
out one of the things that made that easier for her:

> I've been told a number of times, and I know you've heard this
> before too, that we don't look sick. You know, no one would
> ever know we have it.

Not thinking about her illness has helped Jessica take a particular attitude
toward her illness. She explained,

> I don't dwell on the fact that I have cancer, and there are times
> when I forget it until someone, you know, sends me something
> or I have to go for an appointment or whatever. I don't get up

every day and say, "I can't do this, I have cancer, you know!"

For Jessica and those like her, having an outward appearance of health to others and oneself makes it possible to start acting as if nothing is going on. They choose not to dwell on their illness, and they may at times genuinely forget about it. Their stance on the matter justifies this forgetting; the person should not dwell on their cancer and should not avoid aspects of living just because they have cancer.

Being in a reasonably stable condition makes this position easier to attain and hold onto, and these are things that may not be available to everyone. However, some can still choose to not think about it and let it consume their life. Lisa explained how she tries this approach:

> I try to go through each day and not think about it every minute. It's not that I don't know. It's always in the back of my mind that my remission will be over at some point, and I'll have to switch medications. And sooner or later, I'm going to die from lung cancer. It's not that I don't know that. I do know that. I just try to go through every day and pretend that it doesn't exist for at least a good portion of the day until it's time to take my pills, and I can't forget.

Lisa is not in denial; she is just choosing a way to deal with the situation. She added,

> I don't ever want to be one of those people who let cancer consume what I have left of my life, and I don't know if that's really denial or not. I think it's more compartmentalizing. I mean there are so many things that I can't do because of how bad my aerobic capacity is with the scars around my lungs. It's like I wish I could travel. I have the money to travel some more, but I can't walk through an airport.

Lisa sees it, but she chooses to think about things differently. She explains,

> Now, I'm coming to grips with the fact that I can go places if I'm careful and if I let them put me in a wheelchair at the

airport when I have to switch planes between gates quickly. Just getting over that was really hard for me. At my age, to have to sit in a wheelchair and have somebody move me from gate to gate because I can't walk that far in time was really hard to deal with. But I finally said forget it. Who cares? I'm never going to see these people again. If that means I can travel a little bit, let me just do it. What do I care?

For Lisa, if you have a shortened life, you should not reduce it further by consuming that precious time thinking about how short it is! It's not that she doesn't know what her illness means; she does. But she just tries to get through each day and uses more of an active and conscious compartmentalization than passive and subconscious denial.

She knows that she will likely die of cancer, which is a prognostic fact. What she described is precisely what people without the disease struggle to understand. They are made to wonder how the person keeps on going and whether they are in denial.

But we are not in denial. We choose to go through our day without thinking about it every single minute.

For some participants, engaging in what is meaningful makes the task of not focusing on the illness more attainable. Michael gave an example:

There's no doubt that having my son around keeps my mind where my mind needs to be, on my family. Right now, I have the right amount of distraction for just continuing living. There's a dark cloud that follows me wherever I go, but it rarely affects me or keeps me from being productive where I need to be, both at work and at home.

His son keeps Michael's mind focused on his family. And he reminds himself that his mind must be focused in certain places and not in others. Having his son around helps him act on what he thinks is right. His son is a bundle of meaning and joy and also a good distraction.

For some participants, moving on is the right thing to choose. Katherine commented on this:

Well, one of the things that we do as a family, we've always done this, we don't dwell on bad things that happen to us. A lot of times when something happens that we are not happy about, what we do as a family is to say, "OK, well, this happened. How are we going to go forward from here?" That's kind of how we've dealt with it: OK, this happened. How are you moving forward?

For Katherine and others, not dwelling on things is a family value. They move forward. It is their family's tradition and who they are. There is a choice: you can move on, or you can choose to stay obsessed with the illness. Katherine holds onto the belief that she has this choice.

For Katherine, it is good to move on, so that is what she chooses to do. Focusing on living without cancer is another strategy that some participants use. Richard explained,

Some days, I feel quite normal, and this treatment that I'm on is so good that I have had days where I forget I have lung cancer. I mean, I never really forget, but there are days where I'm like, you know, I'm solely focusing on the people who are living, the people who have a life without lung cancer or any cancer, and I will have days just like them.

Richard has days when he forgets about cancer, which is understandable with current treatments that, at least for some, have few or no side effects. And some may argue that there is no utility in dwelling on the illness. It is OK to forget at times. On some days, Richard feels normal and forgets about his cancer, so he carries on living as if nothing matters.

It is OK to sometimes forget about cancer and people with cancer.

Redirecting attention

Redirecting your attention means shifting it away from what is painful or feels useless, and toward what is more useful or meaningful. Larry described this:

In my career, I've had to deal with a lot of uncertainty, and for a large block of time, so I guess I learned that focusing on things that you can control is a lot more productive than focusing on things you can't control. I just learned to accept that. With cancer, I know that there are a great number of uncertainties. I know that I can't change those things and so I don't focus on them. I don't let them drive me crazy.

Larry has dealt with uncertainty often in his career, and he is used to it. He accepts the unknown as part of our condition and doesn't deal with what he cannot change. He focuses on the things that are within his control and finds that to be more productive than focusing on what he cannot control.

There is substantial uncertainty, no doubt, but that cannot be changed. For Larry, people should only focus on what they have the ability to change. Because he knows he cannot change the other aspects, he chooses not to focus on them. Larry added more thoughts:

I have a belief that it doesn't make any sense to worry about things you can't change. I do not sit and worry about the consequences of the disease. I've spent my time doing things. I prefer to do something rather than sit and worry. I have had to deal with a fair amount of uncertainty professionally as a startup company in uncharted territory, and there are only so many hours a day for focusing in on the areas where you can make a difference and be productive. Worrying about things you can't change is a waste of time. That's built into me. It's not something that I necessarily grew out of the box.

In his career, Larry has had to deal with a lot of uncertainty, and he has learned that focusing on things that are within your control is a lot more productive. He learned to accept that and to deal with it. And he doesn't let the things he can't control drive him crazy. He is a person of agency, and that is an essential part of his identity.

Similarly, some participants work on redirecting their attention away from their fear of the worst. Debora uses this coping mechanism:

I try to redirect my attention to something like quilting, or I get involved with folks, so something else I put quilting or creating something. I may watch something on TV; I might go out for a walk and breathe in the air to try to chill out.

Still, it's hard, and the concerns are always there. Debora explained,

I always feel like there's that gun to my head. I fear cancer will again stick its ugly head up and grab my body quickly, and then I'm gone. I don't know how long, I know that the odds are against my survival, and the longer I survive with cancer, the more the odds are against me.

Regardless, Debora keeps reminding herself to stay in the moment. When her mind often starts to wander, she has found it helpful to direct her attention to something that she is doing there and then, such as reading or actively doing something else.

You feel the gun pointed to your head. And you avoid thinking about it by looking somewhere else or feeling something else.

Trying to be positive

Trying to be positive is something that came up often during these conversations. Mary talked about trying to stay positive:

Since I first got diagnosed, I have always tried to stay very positive. I have always said it is what it is. Everybody has their own shit that they deal with. My problems are not any better or any worse than what somebody else might have. I try not to bother with things, and I am just living a more meaningful life. That has helped me with my emotional aspect, although I have found that the filter on my mouth has dissolved since learning I have this. I have a hard time with people who want to fret about things and make big deals about nothing.

Mary tries to be positive. One way she does that is by looking at other people's problems so she can realize that her issues are not any worse or better than someone else's.

One dilemma that can develop for people dealing with serious health issues, however, is an inability to empathize with people struggling with matters that seem less serious. And because we are talking here not about objective facts but rather about evaluative judgments, tensions can develop.

The person with cancer may be happy and content that they are alive and able to spend time with family. Other family members may be bothered that someone arrived late or spilled the milk.

Having these different evaluative frameworks is what can sometimes alienate the person with cancer. Those who fret over what seem like little things, who value things differently, pose a challenge. They may also be a reminder of a privileged world view that is gone and no longer attainable for the person with cancer.

With these thoughts, I am trying to invite reflection. Still, everyone is entitled to their frame of reference and their evaluative judgments. All people are allowed to change their evaluative framework when one does not work well. Each person is also entitled to shun those who are not on the same evaluative page. Further, they are entitled to want to stay positive, optimistic, and not focused on the struggle.

Being positive also takes effort, which is briefly explained by Kim when she says, "As far as day-to-day, just trying to be positive." It is something the person tries to attain and not something that is achieved and then done with. That is also what Donna says: "I try to have a positive attitude in life, and I really try to approach this the same way." These people do not claim that this is a finished project. Yet, they recognize that it is good to have a positive attitude. Some also find the positivity in the diagnosis itself and not only while dealing with the condition. Sharon explained that "I've been able to take advantage of lots of opportunities to find some positivity in the diagnosis." She is making the case that there is positivity to be found in cancer.

Staying positive, like any other coping strategy, has a range and limit. At times, although the person wants to be positive, they recognize the struggle that lies with a heavy weight on their soul. Amy gave voice to this:

I'm staying positive, and we're doing a lot of research, and I have a lot of appointments. So I felt like I was getting back on my feet, I started to do better, and then I got cut down at the knees. It's now . . . everything is up in the air, and it's similar to the feeling of the initial diagnosis. But the difference is at least now I have so much more knowledge. I have so many more connections. I have so much more support. That's what's helping me cope at this point, but when I sit still and think about it, I cry.

Amy is still generally positive and doing what she can to find connection and support. But she has a recurrence, and things are up in the air. Progression of the disease challenges certainty and brings the person down. So while she is trying to be positive, she may have reached the limits of her capacity.

Some participants are determined to continue the fight. For these people, there is one choice and one strategy only, and that is that. Andrew described it:

That's one way I deal with it is to say I'm going to continue to fight, and I'm going to do it. I sometimes think about how my mother survived. She didn't die of cancer. She had colon cancer, and people didn't survive more than a year with or without chemo. We got a second opinion, we learned about a new treatment that was only available in another city, and it was a certain kind of surgery. She had it done when she was eighty-two years old. Here's a woman who could have just laid down and said, "I'm done!" But she didn't. By God, she wanted to live, and she had that surgery done. It was hell on earth for her, but she survived it. She ended up with a colostomy later, very little gut, but she ran a bed and breakfast in a small town for the last four years of her life. And she had to have intravenous fluids two hours a day. She did them, and she just pushed around the IV bag while she did everything else. For her, that cancer was just an irritation because she was living. My mother did not think about dying. She thought about living, and she lived right up to the day she died.

Andrew will continue to fight as his mother did before him. His mother did everything she could, and Andrew wants to do things exactly like her. People have a choice, Andrew makes the case, in how they deal with their cancer. He has the determination to continue the fight, and he has his mother as an inspirational example.

Holding onto faith

Some participants are leveraging coping frameworks that include the infinite. It is through devotional and prayers that they invite divine intervention and maintain a connection with what is beyond. For Kim, coping involves practicing her rituals or having those rituals practiced for her. She was born and raised Catholic, and she is "very devout." She is involved with her church and goes to Mass every day. She prays daily for at least half an hour in addition to going to Mass. She shared,

> One of the first things I did when I was diagnosed was I asked my husband to call our priest and have him perform an anointing of the sick. It is like healing prayers.

Since her diagnosis, she has been to four healing Masses. She explains that these healing ceremonies are just like a regular service, but at the end of the service, the priest or laypeople in the church or deacons will perform healing on each person.

I felt privileged to hear about the experience, which was foreign to me. I realized that this is meaningful to her and that it is important. Furthermore, she believes that it helps her. She is clearly being helped by it. And it is one coping strategy.

For Kim, this is not a new thing. She explained,

> I go to church daily, but I've always been very religious, so this is not a new thing that I started. I've always been a daily Mass goer. So I'm still doing that.

Kim is religious, and that has not changed with the experience of illness. Faith comes to serve when the person is struggling in the day-to-day. When

I asked about how she copes with the anxiety and fears, Kim replied, "I usually try to distract myself, or I pray; I just say a quick prayer."

She prays when she is in distress and prayers do distract.

Kim was not the only one reporting finding help that way. Rebecca shared that she continued going to church and that it helped her mentally. She referred to something she finds that many people agree with her on, which is that simply going to church helps some people.

It was similar with Amanda's practice. Amanda explained that she and her husband attend church regularly:

> My husband and I attend services at our congregation on a pretty regular basis. It gives me a time to reflect and be at peace and be thankful that I can continue to live in the manner which I choose. I feel good and happy about that.

Services give them time to reflect and be at peace. I understand when someone asserts that they live in a manner they choose, and I also understand what they mean when they say that living in this manner makes them happy.

However, these spiritual and ritual practices were not limited to people who identified as religious. Some of the ones who considered themselves nonreligious also shared some about a spiritual dimension. That was the case with Sarah, who hesitantly shared about her experiences with spiritual healers, saying to me, "I don't talk to everybody about it because some people think it's kind of voodoo, but you're a scientist, so take it as you will."

Sarah became open to working with healers. She calls them "spiritual healers" or "body healers." She felt she was opening up her mind to other possibilities. She has worked with multiple healers, and everyone does something different. She pays between one hundred and a few hundred dollars, but she considers that to be an investment in her health. She learned about this in a documentary in which "normal common people, getting in the connection of mind and body, spirits dual connection and healing themselves, like spontaneous remission and spontaneous healing." She discovered that she knows a friend who works for one of the men featured in the documentary. She described what he does:

He's a hands-on healer. He will get into your spiritual energy and pull up those roots of whatever is causing your illness. You sit with a group of people in a small room. They have massage tables. So, people will come in and lie down. It's a very calm and soothing environment, with candles and music. He walks around and lays hands on everybody throughout the process.

Sarah finds this helpful. She recognizes that she spends a significant amount of money on this. Still, she recommends this practice to those who want to find things outside of the box.

Humor

Humor is a coping strategy that many participants use. Amy discussed how she applies humor to cope:

I never let go of my sense of humor. I feel like that has helped keep me sane. It helped mainstream me. It helped me continue to connect with people who are not going through what I'm going through, because there's still a commonality. I keep my laughter and my huge sense of humor and my likeness. I try to hold onto it for dear life, because once you lose that, you set yourself apart. It's like putting yourself in prison. People don't understand why you are so guarded and shut down, and most people don't even care. They look the other way. But if you can stay in touch with your true essence, your true nature and allow that to continue to flourish in the face of this adversity, you connect with humankind, with the world, and that makes a huge difference for me, daily. I don't see many people because of where we live, which is unfortunate because I feel very isolated. But, at least when I speak with people on the phone, or once in a while do FaceTime, I feel that people are leaning in, and they're not kidding me, they're supporting me. That's such a blessing. I don't want to drain anyone, and I don't need pity. What I do need is support, and what I need every day is a few good laughs.

She kept her laughter even as she was saying that to me. Keeping her sense of humor has kept Amy going and helped her stay connected with people.

Humor keeps Amy closer to people and prevents her from becoming alienated. You stay connected when you can still laugh, and this is existentially related to who we are as humans. For people like Amy, pity is not what they want. They want support and a few good laughs every day. And they can tell the difference when what is given is not what they want.

I was amazed at the notion of "mainstreaming someone," and to me, cancer is an alienating disease that disconnects the person from others.

The antidote to cancer is humor. Humor connects the person back to others and draws others in to the person.

Living Life in the Here and Now

For some, coping is about making memories with their loved ones or doing things that are enjoyable to them. This means traveling more for Elizabeth, who explained,

> Now all I want to do is travel because I don't know how much time I have, and I want to make memories with the kids, so that's the other thing is we've just been doing things.

She and her family did not travel much before. People make memories when they travel, and she wants to go places to make memories with her family. She also wants to do the day-to-day things when she can. She became determined not to put things off anymore and to just do them today. Tomorrow may never come. She explained,

> I am doing the things that I put off and said, OK, one day, I'll get to it! I am no longer put that stuff off. We take trips if we have time. Most are driving trips at the spur of the moment. Taking a weekend, getting in the car, and doing something like that, I would never have done that in the past. I would have had it planned out for a long time or put it off entirely. Now we are just not putting that stuff off anymore. We are doing stuff, getting out of the house, just living life, and doing the day-to-day stuff. Because one of the worst things was when I came home from the hospital, and for a good two months, I was in bed or on so many narcotics and still in pain. It took me a long time to wean off the drugs from the initial hospital visit and to feel better with the pain, but I couldn't drive on the narcotics. I couldn't run errands.

Elizabeth started to do the things that she had put off. She travels more with her family because she came to realize that it is not good to put stuff off when there's a real chance the time will come that she can no longer do what she wants.

Coping by connecting with the here and now and by finding one's authentic self resonated with Robert. He broached this topic:

> So immediately, I did a lot of spiritual work, and I wanted to come clean to myself about all the things in my past. I wanted them to have a true love for myself so that I could start healing properly, because something told me that I wasn't going to heal if I did not get all these things in order. Some people say the cancer diagnosis led them to find their authentic self. It is completely true. My diagnosis has led me to myself, and it's like an epiphany. I think I'm not the only cancer person who goes through where you immediately know what is important and what is not, you know? I needed to heal. So anytime I have any self-deprecating thoughts or any self-doubt creeps in, I now redirect them as they come, without any panic or any doubt. I see the thought, and I let it go. I do feel this is helping me to heal in a lot of ways.

Robert wanted to come clean to himself and truly love himself. Cancer led him to himself, and he realized that it is good to first heal, and then it is vital to find authenticity. His way of coping is doing what is truly him.

Doing art work is another coping strategy that keeps the person grounded in the here and now. Samantha explained,

> If I'm feeling down, I go do some art. I've always been an artist. I can't do the same kind of art I used to because my hand is not working, and I can't draw anymore. But I have invented new things, and that's a lot of what I would like to do anyway. I mess around to come up with something new that I might not have thought of before. It is a distraction as much as anything. I don't always come up with something that somebody else will love or that even I will love, but just the messing around with it helps me take my mind off of things. I get in a different brainwave pattern, and it's relaxing. Sometimes I actually think I've come up with something kind of cool, too.

Samantha's hand is not working the way it used to because of brain metastases and treatment. But when she feels down, doing art of any sort helps get her mind off the painful struggle. Even if it is just messing around with objects, art helps because it is not about the pain; it is about the act of expressing.

Music is another tool for coping. Samantha also spoke about music as helpful:

> Music has just been a part of my life forever. I have always had music playing, from the time I was a little girl. My dad was a musician, and we always had music in the house. I'm not a musician, but I always have music in the house. It just helps me feel at home and that I belong. I don't know how to describe it. It's just part of being at peace.

Listening to music helps many patients tremendously.

———————————

Some participants cope by carrying on and continuing with life as it was before diagnosis. Carrying on is attainable for some who have the capacity to still do things almost the same as before cancer. Larry explained,

> My symptoms have been relatively mild compared to what I've seen other people go through. So to a large degree, my life has been rather normal. Most people do not know I have cancer unless I tell them. So, I continue to row. I rowed this summer and every year prior to this, although I row slower and slower. I went to the men's nationals in 2013, and I rowed very poorly, but there was an open-door policy, so I went.

Because his symptoms are mild, he has continued to do what he used to do, albeit a bit less vigorously. He allows himself to row slower. It is OK to row slower. Most important, though, is to keep on rowing. He is accepting this change, although not without some struggle.

Some participants try to maintain normalcy even though life is not what it used to be. Samantha discussed this point of view:

Well, I try to keep a normal life. I'm not working anymore, so we live out in the country. We have a beautiful home, and it's in a beautiful setting, so I can hike. I have a little cabin that sits on that edge of a nearby river, and I walk down there. It's on our property, and it's about a five-minute walk to it. I go down there, and I sit and watch the river. I listen to music a lot. I'm a real music addict. I do yoga, I do art, and I cook still. I'm able to do light housework to keep our house. I have a solarium attached to the house, so I can go out and tend my plants; I do spend quite a bit of time there. I have dogs and a cat, and I enjoy them. My grandson, who's three, lives nearby, and so I see my daughter and her husband and my grandson quite a bit. I have quite a few friends, and I visit with them. Let's see. I try to keep a good attitude. I mean, I try not to think about it as much as I can. I mean, it steals my joy, that's the main thing about having cancer. I can never totally find joy in anything because it's always lurking, but as far as the day-to-day stuff, I still find happiness and peace, and that's how I cope.

In some cases, it is as though joy has been stolen forever. It is lost innocence that will never be recovered or established again. While they keep as much semblance of a normal life as possible, cancer steals the joy for these people, and that always lurks. They can be happy at times, and content, but they can never experience joy the same way again.

Some participants can say that they live in the same way as before. Linda replied,

Honestly, I don't live differently now that I did before. I had to focus in my life on healthy eating and healthy living, being present in my space. You know I feel like all the things that I think would be good for me to do for cancer I was doing before I was diagnosed. So it doesn't feel like I'm doing those things because I have cancer. Does that make sense?

Yet other participants just want to do the normal things that other people take for granted because they have lost them for a while, and they became aware they would eventually lose them entirely. Elizabeth explained this:

> My true help is just to live life. It's not that I forget that I have cancer or pretend that I don't have cancer, but I just continue my day like I did before I had cancer. So I get up, I get the kids ready, I make breakfast, and I do whatever the day needs to do with the kids, get them to their activities. Not to say that I don't have help. I have help, and I have hired sitters to help me. If I am really fatigued, I have people come in and help me. The family helps. But when I can do stuff, I do whatever I can. I feel better if I take the dog for a walk. That's therapeutic. After my cancer diagnosis, all I wanted to do was go to the grocery store, pick up my kids, and take them to their activities. Things that most people are like, "Oh, I'd better do this stuff." That's all I wanted to do because it was taken away from me and it wasn't my choice. Now I love doing those things, the day-to-day stuff. It just keeps me going, and I forget that I'm also a Stage 4 lung cancer patient because I'm busy, and I'm doing things and living life. That has been the best mental thing for me is to just keep going like whether it's there or not, life goes on, and the kids' lives go on, and I've noticed that if I am OK, the family is OK.

Elizabeth does not pretend that she doesn't have cancer, but she continues her days as before. Her real help is to live life.

For participants who lost some abilities, coping is done by trying to start again and do little things. It is through training oneself to do a little and then a little more over time. Nancy spoke about this experience:

> I just recently started working again, kind of freelance, which has been really good for me. I get up and have coffee so I can stay awake and have some energy. I honestly feel like I don't have much of a life right now; I don't have a schedule. I'll try to make myself some food; I will watch TV or I will do some things around the house. If I do that, it takes all my energy. I do try to plan some things. I will be like, OK, I know I'm

getting lunch on a Wednesday with my friends. So, I will take it easy on Monday and Tuesday. Otherwise, on Wednesday, I won't have the energy to go. It is very stressful always trying to monitor my activity level, monitor my fatigue, and I'm always worried that I'm going to have to cancel plans and do that so often.

While Nancy has to monitor her activity level to avoid draining her energy by doing too much, she does not have a set schedule, so she can start by doing little things and train herself to do more.

Resting

Another important way to cope with cancer is to rest when you are tired. Nancy explains this aspect of living with cancer:

> The last couple of months, I've been working, which is so good for me, and it gives me kind of a purpose, a reason to get up. But sometimes I have to call in a day off. But they know me well. I've worked with them for ten years. So, I only say, "I'm having a bad day. I can barely function today," and they go, "Not a problem, we'll handle it." Lately, I will get up and work for a few hours. Then I will rest. I will take a nap in the afternoon. If I don't, I can't even function in the evening. So I will take a nap or at least put my feet up and close my eyes, usually for a few hours. I'll try to eat something healthy, and then I go to bed.

Sometimes, the person has difficult days, and they need more rest. And that is OK. It is OK to rest when tired. Some participants realized that they need to take it easy, and that is how they cope. Lisa agreed, saying she tries to take it easy on herself. There are difficult days, and on those days, you sometimes do not want to do anything. Cynthia remarked,

> There are days when I just think, you know what? I don't feel like even going outside today. I'll just stay in my pajamas and curl up in bed with a good book. That is how I'm coping.

There are days when the person wants to stay in their pajamas and not do anything. One learns to forgive oneself. The coping comes in accepting that you do not need to do certain things in a certain way, you can give yourself some slack.

Pajama days are good, too.

Some realize that they get tired quickly, and with their illness, they allow themselves to take a break. Emily gets fatigued easily, and that is why she is setting limits. She is announcing to others when she is tired. She came to realize that she is not bouncing back as fast as she used to, and she knows that tiring more quickly is not her usual self:

> Well, I was always the toughest member of my family. My husband is very lovely and terrific, but he would be like, "Oh my gosh, I'm so stressed out, I have to go finish my article." I was always bulletproof, a person able to add one more thing and just sleep a bit. I notice now that I'm not rebounding as fast, and if I get overtired one day, I can push it one more day, but then I'm just really, really exhausted and useless for several days after that.

Emily is learning to deal with this. She explained,

> So I'm just setting better limits and saying, "You know what? No. I'm tired, and I have to go take a nap," or "I have to sleep," or "I'm going to take two minutes and prepare a meal that I'm also going to eat."

She recognizes the privilege in relation to her job. She can take some time off and focus on her health and well-being. She explained,

> That's the bonus of my job, right? Humanities professors don't have a lab, and our contract is actually a nine-month contract. I think that's a fallacy because you don't do your research output unless you spend the summer in the archives and do significant writing, but I think I'm just not going to make my promotion. I just will not have the article output that I want to have. If I make it to my next review, I just won't get a promotion. I mean, that's fine.

It is OK to not get the promotion. Emily realizes that she had pride in being the toughest member of the family. But now she is tired more.

When you are tired, you are entitled to rest, and it is perfectly fine. Let those who want the fast track have it. One coping strategy is to be content with the slower track. Emily explained her perspective on her work:

> I would love to finish my book because I like my research and
> I'm interested in it.

Emily is in a work culture where her colleagues check themselves into a hotel for six weeks over the summer after turning their kids over to their parents. That's not possible for her. She does not have the family support she wishes she had. And she is also a hands-on parent. She is now back to working three to five hours a day. She had the option of pushing through in the summer to finish her book, but then everything else would have to get pushed aside. She remarked,

> It feels like there's going to be this huge loss for the people in
> my life, for my family. To say to them, in preparation for that
> loss, "I'm going to focus on this work completely," is not what
> I wanted to do.

Emily had to slow down. She didn't want to be away from her family. Doing that work would mean she couldn't focus on her family as much as she wanted to, which would be a loss for her. If she would have pursued writing her book, then she would have had to sacrifice other valuable things. It is important to write, but it is also important to be a good parent. When the two come into conflict with one another, finishing the book is not as important as being with family. She already gets less clearer hours in the day because of the medications' side effects, especially the fatigue. So, with all her life's constraints, she made a decision:

I've taken this slow. I have taken the slow train.

How Do I Cope?

It was two days after my diagnosis when I'd finished a follow-up imaging of my chest and then went home. I was physically exhausted and emotionally tired. I was lying down and starting to surrender to what I then thought was my fate. I had not yet met my oncologist and knew very little about my condition other than that it was Stage 4 (likely) lung cancer.

A friend of a friend, Hakim, then reached out to me. He was a lung cancer patient himself. He told me exactly what I needed to do: you get your genetic tests as fast as you can, you seek second opinions, and you do all that is in your capacity to keep going.

Hakim, whom I later met once in person, survived years with lung cancer. He had gone through everything. At that time, he had developed over fifteen brain metastases, and he was still fighting. I felt ashamed of wanting to give up before I even started to deal with the problem at hand.

Hakim set the tone for my experience. He is no longer among us, and I wish I would have thanked him enough.

I did not think everything would be all right and could not hold onto positivity. I had my moments of doubts, and I had my moments of despair. I was dreading what I was living. I still feel anxious when things appear to not be going well.

But I wanted to carry on.

It is easy to look back now and think of how I found meaning in the experience and how I was able to do good things. But in complete honesty, cancer sucks, and it is a nasty disease.

I wish I did not have to deal with it, and I do not wish it on any person.

My struggle with the disease early on was in the shifts in my identity and my life prospects. I could not work, and I didn't know how long I would live. My work as a doctor, teacher, and researcher was essential to me. I was also pursuing more academic training so I could do meaningful and useful work in the future. My struggle was when I had to take time off work to deal with my health and when I did not know how I would fare in the future.

I announced my illness to my family and friends. I also shared it with everyone on Facebook. I didn't want people to not know. I felt fortunate to have been able to read what people said about me. I felt like the dead man who can listen to those speaking at his funeral. People did treat me as if I was dying. Many came out of nowhere to say the kindest things. Others also came to give me guidance to the "Right Path," and those were annoying, for sure.

Then after the presidential election, refugees were banned from entering the United States. I thought people must be misguided to believe that refugees, victims of atrocities and horrible war, were coming after us here in the United States with harmful intentions. Having a safe place for refugees and asylum seekers is, I believe, a human right. It was a horrible time in our history.

I believed I could do something about it. If I came out and let people look at the face of the unknown people who suffer, maybe they would better understand. Maybe if people heard my story, they could start to understand the impact of these horrid policies on the lives of people who are human, just like them. In the end, I was a doctor and a professor here at an American university. In all my work, I was serving the community, whether that was by taking care of patients myself or by teaching the doctors who would take care of those patients.

I went public with my story and shared my experience and how the ban affected me personally as, at that time, it made it harder for me to see some of my siblings while I was struggling with advanced cancer. My story got the attention of a broad audience, but then it started to metamorphose. I wanted to keep hold of my narrative, so I wrote a *Huffington Post* letter to the president that helped me reclaim my voice and reconstruct my identity.

Now I am not only a doctor, researcher, and teacher. I am also a patient. I reconciled with being vulnerable. I accepted being what I am. Most importantly, I claimed an authentic voice that is not afraid of speaking truth to power.

I was fortunate enough to be able to go back to work soon after that experience. I was able to build my work schedule gradually, and I returned to seeing patients and teaching. I had an urgency to complete some of the research work I was doing and to finish my PhD dissertation. I defended that last year (2018), and it was great to do so.

In returning to being a doctor again, I brought my perspectives and insights I'd gained as a patient. I became curious about the patient as a person, about their lives and how their illnesses impact them. I became better at listening and understanding. I wanted to turn my interactions with patients into spaces for them to reflect on what is important for them in their health and to find ways that work for them to get where they wished to be. It was important for me to do a good job as a doctor. My sensitivity to cancer has now probably helped me uncover at least two cases of cancer that had been previously overlooked because of vague presentations.

I coped with my illness by engaging in reflections and dialogues. I wanted conversations with people. I wanted to share, and I wanted to listen. I also wanted to reflect and understand myself. I attended therapy for a few months, and it was helpful to some extent. I also practiced reflective writing. I would say that my writing, whether for the scholarly work I've published or the reflective pieces that build on my own experiences, were critical in helping me make sense of my experience. I still also find my conversations with others to be the most meaningful things I do, and I am developing my capacity to mentor others by bringing to bear my experiences as a person and as a scholar. I have shared my story, and I am using my insights in broader conversations so that others can reflect on their stories and bring their authentic experiences to the conversations.

When I think of coping, music also comes to mind. I am speaking here particularly about one album: *Hamilton*. I owe Lin-Manuel Miranda a lot, because his work had an enormous impact on my experience. When I went to see the musical the first time with Crystal, I cried throughout most of the songs. I ran to the bathroom to cry more and wash my face afterward, and I could not speak a word for the rest of the night.

But in a few days, Crystal and I were able to listen to all of the songs again together and to reflect on each one. From then until today, the album has been my favorite.

I relate to the experience of the immigrant who did not take for granted that he would be alive. It was very salient in my mind that this is my one and only shot. So my primary way of coping had been by writing, and I was running out of time. I also did not know who, other than me, would tell my story, if anyone. Most importantly, I was struggling to allow myself to love and be loved while cancer has been my reality. I was with the woman who was witnessing the scenes acted on the stage and is witnessing me as a play of destiny.

Hamilton pushed my reflection into raw spaces, but also helped me heal.

However, I would say my number one coping mechanism was doing this very work. I learned so much from each person I interviewed. Every person challenged me. My capacity to be open, permeable, and understanding was developed and used to its limit. I would not deny that the experience was extremely painful. It was traumatizing and retraumatizing. It was as if I tore open a wound each time it started to heal. It was also fatiguing and, at times, frightening. In the beginning, I would do two interviews in one day. But then, I could not do more than one every few days. It would take me days to recover and heal again. To open oneself up to the pain is excruciating for the body but enlightening for the soul. It was worth every minute, every tear, and every sigh.

I could not be more grateful to those who allowed me into their personal spaces and shared their stories with me.

I was honored.

One of my existential answers to the problem of my death was to write a book that can live on someone's shelf after I die. I want it to be in philosophy and to sit next to Hegel's work or next to Kant's or Habermas's. I do not really know if that would ever happen. I do not know if I would be given the time to learn enough, to think enough, to converse with enough people, and to write a masterpiece.

I do not know.

The only thing I know is that I am determined to work as much as I can to transcend my limits. If my time comes before doing something meaningful for others, I will know that I have given it my best.

I also know that the work could be developed more with more edits and rewriting. But I am sending this out as it stands now because I am running out of time and need to start on the next project.

I will always be working on writing, editing, and rewriting the narrative.

What else can I do to cope better?

I could use more good laughs. I could also breathe deeper.

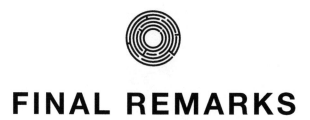

FINAL REMARKS

I will end this book with a few reflections and remarks. These are what I hope my reader has noticed in these pages.

No one is an exception, and no one is immune from cancer, this nasty disease. Many people have gotten it; you could get it, too! The forty people whose stories are in this book are making meaning and building resilience while living with these incurable cancers, and so can everyone else. Many of us in this book have privileges that made it possible to find the diagnosis early enough and to receive treatment that has kept us alive for some time. But, by the time you read these words, many of us will be gone. What will be left are memories in the minds of those who loved us, our deeds, and these stories.

I wrote this book as one answer to my existential struggle. I also wrote it to open space for others to advance the conversations around their existential inquiries. The answer I have proposed implicitly and explicitly in this work, the same that many of these participants also suggested, is simple. You can deal better with your existential struggle if you do not obsess about it and, instead, pay attention to others' struggles. It is when a person shifts their mind from worrying about their own aches and opens their soul to empathize with the suffering of others that they can transcend their limits and their existential fears.

But it is not all about fear. These are forty stories of hope. Yes, we live at a time when there is plenty of hope for those still living with lung cancer. At the same time, there is a lot of work yet to be done. Now, these people are living longer, and the question is how to make their lives more tolerable, more fulfilled, and more enjoyable. There is a lot to be done.

Cancer is an isolating disease. It is isolating because it is not understood, by the patient or by others. The person who has cancer suffers alone, even when people are around. There is a lot to be done to break this pattern of isolation. For instance, let's open spaces for patients with cancer to continue to live in the mainstream of life and not be shoved to the margins.

When you develop cancer, you will have an identity crisis. I guarantee that. There is a discontinuity, and the person is not the same as before. The good news is that many people can reconstruct their identity and keep going. And the person can keep going without living with loss. But the opposite can also be true. The person could continue on with access to added meaning having had an awakening.

The stories here are of ordinary people, just like you and me. I wrote the stories for ordinary people, just like you and me. The average person, whether living unseen or living on the margin of the scene, has many rich stories that are worth being told. These stories are worth hearing. We can learn tons from those who struggle with cancer and live at the limits of time. We can learn about who we are, and we can reflect on who we will become if faced with a similar threat. Tarrying at the limits of time is a privileged position of enlightenment and insight.

But still, people with lung cancer are suffering every day. They are misunderstood, and their experiences are mischaracterized. There is still the stigma around lung cancer with its relationship to smoking, and that sucks. It sucks, and it sucks badly to be blamed for a disease you are suffering from that you played no role in creating. It sucks when you have been forbidden empathy because you are blamed for your illness. Humans can only do so much, and our control over our destiny is finite. We deserve care from one another, and that, conversely, *can* be unlimited.

Patients with cancer need support in finding meaning while living life and dealing with mundane day-to-day concerns. They also need understanding as they struggle to make sense of their illness. They deserve spaces to support them as they redefine who they are and continue to author their narratives. They also deserve listening ears when they explain why and how they feel or struggle with this or that feeling or constraint. Still, you should not expect that you can find the meaning for them. They may not find it themselves, either, and that is OK. Our life projects may never be finished while we are still alive.

When the person searches for meaning, they might choose to elaborate whatever philosophies or frameworks they fancy, or they could opt to live life in the here and now. There is no one answer for every person's question. There is no one "why." No one story explains us all. Yes, there is meaning in knowing and learning. There is meaning also in relationship, connectedness, and community. There is a lot of meaning in living for a purpose and transcending one's limits by being there for others. But there is meaning in not searching for any meaning and just simply living. There is also a choice of rejecting the notion of meaning altogether.

Within this or that framework of viewing life, cancer is still a significant adversity. But people do build resilience if they are granted the right conditions. Some people are more fortunate than others in terms of their predisposition for being resilient as, drawing on their previous life, they strive to live with the cancer better. People can make it easier for the patient to develop strength if they give the right support. The person cannot do it alone.

Knowledge empowers patients to deal with the uncertainty and to have hope. But at times, some will feel the need to reach beyond, into religion, to find strength, and that is all right, too. It is also OK to not be strong, and it is OK to feel broken. The person should be able to say, "I am broken inside and cannot do it anymore." They can also choose to keep on until they can no longer keep on.

All of society should be part of making the experience of the ill tolerable. That should be what defines us as humans. But especially with those who work in health care, it is their duty because they made a commitment to taking care of others. Providing experiences with health care that are supportive of autonomy and respectful of patients' perspectives are essential. In the end, people do what they want to do.

In reality, people do all kinds of health actions. For me, as a physician, it is good to be doing what is useful and avoiding what is not. But it is OK for someone else to do what they want as long as it is not preventing them from doing what is useful for their wish to attain some desired effect. Otherwise, they are not doing what is in their best interest. And yes, the targeted chemotherapy medicines work and are good at keeping people alive. It is likely to not be turmeric or ginger that is healing people but rather the medicines, which have been proven to work.

Whether I agree with the patients' practices or not, my commitment is to listen to what people want to do and why they want to do what they are doing. Doctors can understand a lot when they talk to people and hear why they do or do not do certain things. As a doctor, I learned from doing these interviews that I should listen more. And I should do it with an open mind and curiosity. I also learned that it is not that people do not know or do not want to do what they think is right. At times, people just *cannot*.

It is suitable for doctors to also know that people do all kinds of things, at times without telling them and even against their recommendations. It could be helpful to open spaces for conversations so people can make better, more informed choices. Also, people make health choices not just because of their life philosophy but also because of specific constraints. Many, many people resort to alternative medicine approaches because they cannot afford visits to medical doctors and the copays that come from the tests medical doctors do, let alone the entire cost of those tests.

People cope using multiple strategies, and many of them work and work well. Cancer is a disease that threatens a person's existence of the self as a person. Thus, maintaining agency is essential for a sense of well-being and for coping. Advocacy, volunteering, mentoring, and participating in research are all noble strategies that leverage the new identity of the person. Cancer then can become an addition that is valued rather than a subtraction. I am a person, and I have cancer. Now I can stand in solidarity with people in ways that were not attainable to me before.

People want to carry on with relationships, but they want to be understood and treated with care and support. Patients with cancer have little space for annoying people, and they are, more than ever, capable of speaking truth and not holding back. If you want to connect with an authentic person who cares about and values quality time, then find a cancer patient. If you are not willing to be mindful, thoughtful, or reflective, then maybe cancer patients are not good friends for you.

People with cancer shift their frames of reference and their priorities. They value things differently. They may feel they are running out of time and have little room for trivial things. This shift in preferences can become a source of stress in their relationships with others. It also makes it harder for them to be understood. That is why support groups are essential. People who have cancer understand one another. Support groups, many people would argue, should be part of the care plan for cancer patients. Counseling and psychotherapy can be good for some people as well. One could say that therapy is useful for all of us at some point or another in life. Who would not want to understand themselves better? Who would not wish to see the world with better mindfulness?

Cancer patients are often too aware of their condition and are not usually in denial. They shift their focus and choose where to direct their attention. People are entitled to choose where they want their focus. They are entitled to describe their experiences and reflect on them within frameworks that make sense to them. Yes, it is hard for the person without cancer to understand. It is hard, however, in part because people may not listen enough. If we allow ourselves to be permeable, then we can see where the person with cancer is coming from.

Living life in the here and now as opposed to thinking about what tomorrow could bring has helped some patients with cancer. It kept them grounded and focused and allowed them to keep on doing what they want to do. Humor also helps those who wanted to stay in the mainstream and maintain connectedness. So, too, did resting help. People with cancer have to renegotiate the economy of their energy so they can continue doing meaningful things.

I have rambled in the past few pages of my reflection on the whole book as I tried to share ideas I want to leave with the reader. If the reader, however, would take one idea and one idea only, my advice is that it be this: I can transcend my limits by doing things for not only *myself* but also for *others*. I want to live and be here as a person, but if I transcend my limits by doing things and genuinely living *for* and *with* my cherished others, then even when I die, I will continue.

The End

References

[1] Rebecca L. Siegel, Kimberly D. Miller, and Ahmedin Jemal, "Cancer Statistics, 2017," CA: Cancer Journal for Clinicians 67, no. 1 (January/February 2017): 7–30, https://doi.org/10.3322/caac.21387.

[2] "Key Statistics for Lung Cancer," American Cancer Society, last modified January 8, 2019, https://www.cancer.org/cancer/non-small-cell-lung-cancer/about/key-statistics.html.

[3] Emily Harrop et al., "Managing, Making Sense of and Finding Meaning in Advanced Illness: A Qualitative Exploration of the Coping and Wellbeing Experiences of Patients with Lung Cancer," Sociology of Health & Illness 39, no. 8 (November 2017): 1448–1464, https://doi.org/10.1111/1467–9566.

[4] Zhao Chen et al., "Non-Small-Cell Lung Cancers: A Heterogeneous Set of Diseases," Nature Reviews: Cancer 14 (July 24, 2014): 535–546, https://doi.org/10.1038/nrc3775.

[5] Ayana Smith, Yolanda M. Hyde, and Deb Stanford, "Supportive Care Needs of Cancer Patients: A Literature Review," Palliative & Supportive Care 13, no. 4 (August 2015): 1013–1017, https://doi.org/10.1017/S1478951514000959.

[6] M.E. Giuliani et al., "The Prevalence and Nature of Supportive Care Needs in Lung Cancer Patients," Current Oncology 23, no. 4 (August 2016): 258–265, https://doi.org/10.3747/co.23.3012.

[7] Phil Francis Carspecken, Critical Ethnography in Educational Research: A Theoretical and Practical Guide (New York: Routledge, 1996).

Made in the USA
Middletown, DE
23 September 2019